HYPNOTHERAPY
Healing Through The Mind

P. Uma Devi

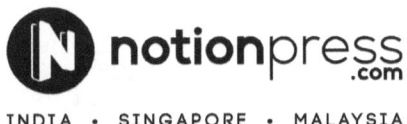

INDIA • SINGAPORE • MALAYSIA

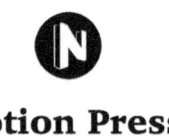

Notion Press

No.8, 3rd Cross Street,
CIT Colony, Mylapore,
Chennai, Tamil Nadu – 600004

First Published by Notion Press 2020
Copyright © P. Uma Devi 2020
All Rights Reserved.

ISBN 978-1-63714-603-3

This book has been published with all efforts taken to make the material error-free after the consent of the author. However, the author and the publisher do not assume and hereby disclaim any liability to any party for any loss, damage, or disruption caused by errors or omissions, whether such errors or omissions result from negligence, accident, or any other cause.

While every effort has been made to avoid any mistake or omission, this publication is being sold on the condition and understanding that neither the author nor the publishers or printers would be liable in any manner to any person by reason of any mistake or omission in this publication or for any action taken or omitted to be taken or advice rendered or accepted on the basis of this work. For any defect in printing or binding the publishers will be liable only to replace the defective copy by another copy of this work then available.

Dedicated to
The Universe and Humanity

…… There is no limit to the power of the human mind. The more concentrated it is, the more power is brought to bear on one point……

Swami Vivekananda

Contents

Foreword   9

Acknowledgements   11

Preface   13

Part I: Fundamentals of Hypnotherapy

Chapter One:	Introduction: My Quest into Hypnotherapy	19
Chapter Two:	Power of the Subconscious Mind	28
Chapter Three:	Hypnosis and Hypnotherapy	34
Chapter Four:	Pre-Induction Interview, its Purpose and Advantages	40
Chapter Five:	Hypnotherapy Session and Post Hypnotic Suggestions	46
Chapter Six:	Emotional Basis of Physical Diseases	52
Chapter Seven:	Visualization and Guided Imagery	59
Chapter Eight:	Self Hypnosis	65
Chapter Nine:	Regression Therapy	71

Part II: Applications of Hypnotherapy

Chapter Ten:	Introduction	81
Chapter Eleven:	Nonclinical Applications	86
Chapter Twelve:	Clinical Applications	110

Chapter Thirteen: Other Areas of Application 130
Chapter Fourteen: Applications in Children 136

Epilogue 161
Further Reading 163
Index of Words 165

Foreword

It is with great happiness that I see this informative book 'Hypnotherapy: Healing through the Mind' coming into the hands of valued seekers of therapy to eliminate the root cause of their issues, written by Dr. P Uma Devi. I have known her for half a century as a friend and a dedicated scientist in Radiation Biology.

She has applied the same methods of scientific enquiry in her practice of this science of 'mind.' You are seeing the result of her learning in this book. She learned 'Clinical Hypnotherapy' after retiring from her illustrious career in Radiation Biology, trying to know the fundamental causes of disease.

Here, Dr. Uma Devi with her more than 15 years of experience of practicing 'Clinical Hypnotherapy' (any therapy performed on a person when she/he is under a state of hypnosis or under an altered state of mind is termed 'hypnotherapy'), brings to the reading public in India and abroad a book written in a very simple language explaining "what is hypnosis and Clinical Hypnotherapy" for the layman.

To support her view that hypnotherapy can be very useful for helping people overcome their mental, emotional, energetic and physical conditions and issues, she has described many cases of her clients (patients) who overcame their disturbing conditions and live a happy cheerful life, free from the cause creating the condition.

She has demystified the term 'hypnosis' as described in the English to local vernacular dictionaries, which has resulted in its misunderstanding in India. The dictionaries confuse the researcher by giving the meaning as 'SammohanVidya or Vashikaran Mantra.' It is not so. Hypnosis is not a

'Tantric' process, it is purely a 'psychological process.' When Dr. Sigmund Freud gave up 'hypnosis,' Dr. Carl Jung, his associate still continued using it in his practice.

In India, ever since Dr. Sunny Satin and I started teaching and practicing 'Clinical Hypnotherapy,' we met many people educated and uneducated who were open to this science of healing through 'the altered state of consciousness/mind.' There were many others who were biased against it, but they also did not take pains to do scientific research, and without enquiry or experiencing themselves would reject it. It does take all types of people to make the world.

I am very happy that Dr. Uma Devi (a person acknowledged internationally in her scientific field) has written a book on Clinical Hypnotherapy for the Indian public with real cases from India. I have read the complete book and recommend it to the readers and seekers of true therapy, without medicine, just working with the mind. Still people should understand that it is not a cure all as for a human there are many other factors causing disease, but a good therapist can help to unravel the cause.

I wish the reading public a very learning time with this book, may you open up to healing yourself by working with your mind.

29.10.2020

Yogesh Choudhary, C. Ht.

Director,
Indian Institute of Hypnotherapy,
Gurugram, India

Acknowledgements

My sincere thanks are due to Dr. Yogesh Choudhary and late Dr. Sunny Satin, Founder of the California Hypnosis Institute, USA, for introducing me to this wonderful subject. I never thought that I can become a hypnotherapist but for the constant encouragement they gave in pursuing the subject. I am highly benefited by the experience gained from the patients and clients who trusted me and came for therapy; I am indebted to them. My students have been a great inspiration to me for exploring more into the depths and the surprises that hypnotherapy holds. I thank them for their active interest and participation in the frequent discussion meetings. My thanks are due to Dr. Yogesh Choudhary for his valuable suggestions in improving the manuscript and for writing the Foreword. I would also like to thank my nephew Shashi Kumar for editing and formatting the manuscript.

Even though I kept it for the last, this is the most important for me; the Superior Power, whatever it may be, for being there to guide me and give the right insights at the right time in the form of thoughts and ideas that have helped me to sail through difficult times and taxing situations smoothly and to learn from those experiences; millions of thanks and salutations to that invisible presence, without which this book would not have been possible.

Preface

When something goes wrong in our life, contrary to expectations, we feel unhappy, frustrated and disappointed. This may be expressed as anger, grief or despair. We start blaming the circumstances, the situation or the people we think are behind it or take it as a punishment for our past misdeeds. The human mind has a tendency to focus on the negatives, making it worse and worse, creating a mindset that sees nothing good or worth living.

If we can take these experiences in a positive manner, realizing that they are the opportunities offered to us for learning and improving, they can form the stepping stones to success and happiness. There is nothing called punishment or failure; they are opportunities to learn from the experience and the tests that we have to take. Every one of us possesses all the resources needed to pass those tests and emerge out with more strength and determination. This is easily achievable by making use of our natural resources in the best possible manner. The only thing one needs to do is to understand that only we, and nobody else, are responsible for creating our experiences and prepare ourselves to face them. Others are there to facilitate this learning process by providing the needed circumstances, giving us the opportunity to discover and use our natural resources. Thus, one has to create the mindset to accept the responsibility for our life experiences and prepare ourselves to face them confidently.

Hypnotherapy helps to create this mindset, generating a positive outlook and proper approach towards our life experiences, especially the seemingly difficult ones. It functions at the mind level, helping us to learn and correct the mistakes and move forward with more understanding of oneself and others, more tolerance and patience, leading to success and happiness.

I have included a number of actual case studies that validate the multifarious uses of hypnotherapy, but the names of the persons are changed to conceal their identity and protect confidentiality.

The names of the persons cited in the actual case studies are changed to conceal their identity and protect confidentiality.

Part I
Fundamentals of Hypnotherapy

Chapter One

Introduction: My Quest into Hypnotherapy

Decisions based on cold reason alone are usually made to satisfy others. Intuitive decisions make us feel good, even if others think we are crazy.

— *Elisabeth Kübler-Ross*

My learning has only started. I am still learning and there is a lot to learn. Human mind is the biggest mystery and a storehouse of surprises. A whole lifetime will not be enough to understand even one-tenth of that mystery. Each patient gives a new experience and an opportunity to learn; and that makes me humbler, realizing how little I know.

My introduction to hypnotherapy was through a friend, Dr. Yogesh Choudhary, a well known hypnotherapist based in Delhi, who used to talk of the wonderful and amazing experiences he had with his patients. He told about the higher souls and Masters, who are ever ready to help us. He talked about the unlimited powers of our subconscious mind and the great possibilities to utilize them for better health, happiness and peace. I, being addicted to experimental research for more than 30 years, was not convinced. But then curiosity overrode my skepticism and I decided to give it a try. I attended the 'Introductory Course' of the California Hypnosis Institute, conducted in Delhi. The course was interesting, and I learned the basic concepts and techniques to hypnotize a willing person and give suggestions under hypnosis. Still I was not very confident or optimistic that it is going to work in my hands. But now I believe that God has His own ways of opening human eyes for a purpose that He has designed for us. It can come in different ways and in my case, it came in the form of a student who needed help. As the Professor and Head of the Department of Research in the Cancer Hospital, Bhopal in Central India, I was guiding doctorate students. One of my Ph.D. students, a young lady of 24 years, was suffering from depression, following the death of her mother from brain cancer. She, being the only child and very attached to her mother, was not able to come out of the trauma. She remained aloof, not mingling with other students, or participating in the usual activities of youngsters of her age. She was gloomy, very quiet and there was no smile to brighten her beautiful face. She wanted to come out of it but felt helpless. I had just returned after doing the basic course and during the tea break, I talked about hypnotherapy and its therapeutic possibilities, how it can help to resolve emotional problems, etc. as was told in our class.

That evening this young lady, let us call her Karuna, came to me. Her face showed anxiety and confusion. She timidly asked me if I can do hypnotherapy on her. I was surprised because I did not think that anybody would allow me to test my new learning on them. I was honest in my reply and told her that even though I have learned the technique, I do not know whether it will work. But if she wants, I shall do it. She was desperate to get back to normal life and was willing to try anything. So, we fixed a time on the following Sunday. The session was to be conducted in my quarters.

Karuna came to my house promptly at the appointed time. After preliminaries, we went to the issue and I gathered the information needed in half hour. She was very low in self-confidence, and her thoughts and feelings were mostly on the negative side. I had learnt that in such cases, suggestions given under hypnosis to build confidence and cultivate positive thinking can be effective. I wrote down a suggestion to release negative feelings and increase self-confidence and make her more positive in attitude and showed it to her; she said it is what she wants. Now we were ready for the actual process. I used a method called the arm raising induction I had learned in the course, to put her into trance, and deepened further by progressive relaxation suggestion. She went quite deep, which meant that her conscious mind had completely withdrawn to the background and her subconscious mind was now open to the therapist's suggestion. I read out the suggestion that I had written and then awakened her. She felt more relaxed, and her face showed it. We did another session after two days, and again a session after another couple of days, every time repeating the same suggestions.

I was in for a surprise! The next week when I was in my office, I heard a peal of laughter from the next room where the students used to gather for snacks and tea. Curiosity took me there and I found Karuna chatting jovially with the other students who were enjoying a joke that she told – the laughter I heard was a part of it. They invited me for a cup of tea, which I gladly accepted. There was an expression of disbelief on many faces at the miraculous change they were seeing in their colleague. They asked me what magic I have done to change her so within a week's time. My thought was also not very different.

That incident really changed my view and I decided to do the full three level course of Hypnotherapy offered by the California Hypnosis Institute. I wanted to become a hypnotherapist and devote my time to alleviate the sufferings of my fellow humans, even at the expense of my research interests, which I do not regret for a moment.

Hypnotherapy is a method of treatment that uses the powers of the subconscious mind for healing. It can be rightly called 'healing through mind.' Access to the subconscious mind is a pre-requisite for the healing. The hypnotherapist uses hypnosis as a tool to reach the subconscious mind. The receptivity of the mind to verbal suggestions increases many-fold during hypnosis; suggestion given in this state is readily accepted and the subconscious mind makes it the reality and it becomes effective. We will go into the details later in the book.

My initial experiences in hypnotherapy came from my students and some cancer patients admitted to the hospital in the terminal stage of disease. The results of pain relief in the cancer patients were unbelievable.

> My first patient was a 15 year old boy, with the disease spread to almost every part of the body, including bone joints, abdominal cavity, and liver. Doctors had given him a maximum of 3 months more to live. He was in terrible pain, unable to eat or sleep. He was too weak to tolerate chemotherapy and was on morphine, taken every 4 hours, and even that was not able to control his pain. When he was brought to me, he had not been able to sleep, even with morphine, for about 3 weeks. Food intake was almost nil, and he was just skin and bones. His knees were swollen, and walking was difficult and very

painful; he was brought in a wheelchair. He was willing to try any treatment that does not involve medication or injection. I made him lie down on a couch and induced hypnosis by progressive relaxation (this is a method which uses suggestions to relax the body and calm down the mind). He went into a deep trance within a few minutes. I gave suggestion to release the feeling of pain and discomfort, followed by another suggestion that he is free from pain and feeling hungry, therefore when he goes back he takes food and goes to sleep, immediately falling asleep and having a sound sleep. Then he was awakened and sent to his hospital ward. To my surprise, after the session he went back walking, without any help. It was about 6 in the evening. Immediately after reaching the ward he had a meal and went off to sleep without taking the morphine dose and slept undisturbed for 4 hours. I did two more sessions on him and he was pain-free and was taken off morphine. But since the disease was in a very advanced stage, he could not survive and died within 3 months. During that period, he was comfortable and cheerful.

Another case of cancer pain was a 72 year old woman, with recurring anal cancer and was on morphine for pain control. She felt hungry, but was afraid to take food, as she shuddered at the thought of going to the toilet. Passing stools and urine was very painful. She was willing to do anything that can relieve the pain and agreed for hypnotherapy. Two sessions gave considerable relief from the pain and the morphine dose was reduced to half; after 4 sessions the pain completely disappeared, and morphine could be stopped. She started taking food without fear and became more cheerful. Though she did not survive long, her remaining days were peaceful and comfortable, and she was taking meals regularly and sleeping without medicines.

These cases show that hypnotherapy can benefit people of any age and can help improving the quality of life even in patients with terminal diseases.

Why Use Hypnotherapy?

Modern approach to ailments is to treat the symptoms using medicines, looking at each problem as a disease of the body or the mind. Even though the treatment may succeed in alleviating the symptoms and apparently restore normal condition, many a time it does not ensure complete health of the person. This is because the treatment methods and medication are generalized in terms of the disease symptoms or behavioral pattern, often ignoring the individual personality – emotional, psychological, and spiritual – that plays a significant role in the treatment response. Therefore, even though the patient is cured in the medical sense, the illness persists, compromising the quality of life. A holistic health approach should take into consideration the body-mind relationship, as most diseases have a mental, emotional, and physical component. In many cases, the physical symptoms may be the bodily reaction to some emotional or mental problem, or even an adverse drug reaction. So, treating the body alone does not give full benefit to the patient.

Hypnotherapy is a method of treatment that makes use of the body-mind relationship for holistic healing. It is built on the concept that mind is at the root of all our issues/problems and nothing can happen without the knowledge of the mind; and can even be created by the mind. If the mind has the power to create a problem, it can also resolve it. As hypnotherapy approaches the mind for the therapeutic movement, medicines do not have any place in the treatment. It is an internal experience, not something that can be explained in words. One must feel it to understand and appreciate it. It is not governed by logic, but intuition plays a role in guiding the therapist; it may come as a thought, an idea or as a feeling, or even from a word or sentence spoken by the patient/client. Therefore, a therapist cannot go by a preconceived program and should be prepared for surprises. A hypnotherapist treats each patient/client as a unique person with his/her own perception and feelings.

Hypnotherapy has generally been found to be very effective in many areas of self-improvement like changing some attitudes and habits, personality development, increasing self confidence and self-esteem, removing anxiety, fears and phobias, and in relieving pain, resolving relationship issues, also in treating chronic diseases like asthma, depression, diabetes, hypertension, psoriasis etc., stop alcoholism, smoking and other addictive habits. This is discussed in more detail later in the book (see Applications of Hypnotherapy). Since many people come to hypnotherapy for resolving non-clinical emotional and behavioral issues rather than clinically diagnosed diseases, in this book they are referred to as clients, not as patients.

Spiritual Basis of Hypnotherapy

> *The future is unconsciously prepared long in advance and therefore can be guessed by clairvoyants.*
>
> – Carl Jung

Hypnotherapy is a spiritual science. We are all spiritual beings, taken birth in human body for the purpose of soul evolution by learning through experience. Earth is considered to be the school for this learning. The lesson to be learned is decided based on 'Karma' that it desires to be liberated from. The karma concept is a part of the Hindu Philosophy, which says that what we experience in this life is a consequence of our deeds in the past lives, but may not be familiar or accepted by other systems of belief.

Before taking birth, the soul plans all the experiences, circumstances, activities, people, relationships, etc. that can help in this learning process and the karma resolution. This plan is made by the soul in consultation with the Higher Self that is a part of the Supreme Spirit or the Creator, and this forms the "Life Script" of the person. When the soul enters the body of the fetus in the womb it brings this script, along with the knowledge and information accumulated through the experiences in the previous lives and is stored in the subconscious memory. What happens after birth is guided by this life script, so nobody else is responsible for the good or bad experiences a person encounters. A soul may take several births for learning different lessons, thereby evolving to higher energy levels, till further incarnations are not needed. The subconscious mind keeps a record of all the experiences of each lifetime that is not accessible to the conscious mind in the present life. The cause of many of our current problems may lie in the past life experiences and can be resolved by going into that memory. Hypnotherapy uses hypnosis to access the subconscious memory and remove the conflicts and negative impressions, accelerating the learning process by resolving the unresolved issues, resulting in catharsis, and healing. The hypnotherapist may assist in this resolving while the client is viewing the past life events.

Why Hypnotherapy is not widely Accepted?

A few days back I received a phone call from a prospective client. He had some problems that his friend said can be resolved by hypnotherapy, but he had apprehensions. So, he called me to clarify his doubts. He wanted to know whether hypnosis is safe and if he will be normal after undergoing hypnotherapy. I get several enquiries like this and raising other fears that clearly express the misconceptions and false image of hypnosis as something dangerous and, therefore, to be avoided. Influence of stage shows and visual media have a big role in creating such an image. People may have seen movies where hypnosis is pictured as some magical process or something like voodoo through which one can bring the person under his control and make him/her do whatever he commands, even robbery and murder. Moreover, the meaning of hypnosis in the vernacular dictionaries are sometimes misleading, e.g. *"Sammohan Kriya (Vidya)"* gives an impression that it is a sort of enchantment that subdues the person into total obedience. Another wrong idea many people entertain is that the hypnotist has some special powers in his/her eyes and can hypnotise somebody by simply looking into the eyes of the person.

Several other misplaced notions exist about hypnotherapy, which do not have any basis. Mostly, they originate from a fear of loss of self-control associated with stage shows. A few instances are there, where a half-baked hypnotist tries to pose as a genuine therapist and treat people with big promises of cure. Gullible clients who are lured by their advertisements can have unpleasant experiences, when they are not able to relax or if they are not awakened properly at the end of the session. Such experiences lead to fear and distrust of hypnotherapy in general. But used in the proper way by a qualified hypnotherapist, this method can work wonders and give long-lasting relief from even problems that have not found success with the conventional methods of therapy.

At this point I want to emphasize that hypnosis is not *"Sammohan"* or enchantment or any tantric rite, but it is a state of deep concentration on one thing to the exclusion of everything else. In that state one can access deep seated memories and get an inner awareness that is not possible in the normal waking state, which can be used to remove disturbing emotions, resolve problems, and bring about mental and physical healing. It is a temporary state and after waking up from hypnosis the person remains absolutely normal.

There are people, usually accompanying a client, a relative or friend of the family, who come thinking that hypnosis will be done in front of the whole group as is seen in the movies, so that they can watch it and tell to others. There was a serial telecast on one of the Hindi channels a few years back, showing some actual cases of past life regression (PLR), as being done by a therapist. To make it more interesting they were showing video clips using actors, along with the audio description of the client's response to the therapist's questions. After watching that, some people asked me to be allowed to sit with the client when I am doing PLR, thinking that they can see the events on a screen. They were disappointed when I told them that only the person under hypnosis can see it on their mental screen, as it is happening in their mind.

One usual question coming from new clients is 'will I be normal after waking up, can I drive, will I need somebody's help to go home?.' The answer is that when a person wakes from hypnosis, he/she feels refreshed and relaxed, like waking up from a good night's sleep.

> After I started practicing hypnotherapy, I visited my friends in Germany, a cancer therapist and his wife. I was their guest. I was talking about hypnotherapy and they were fascinated by it. Next evening when he came back from the hospital, he said it was a heavy day, there were several new patients and he was very tired. I asked him if he wants to relax fast through hypnosis. He was enthusiastic about the idea. He went easily into deep hypnosis. I gave suggestion to release stress and go into deep relaxation, and then woke him up. He felt so refreshed that he immediately went out and practiced for a marathon run he was participating the next week.

Some people have a fear of getting stuck in hypnosis. Hypnotherapy is being practiced in several countries for many years now and nobody is known to get stuck in hypnosis. During my 15 years of practice I never had an experience of anyone stuck in hypnosis. Sometimes a person may slip into natural sleep and then will wake up to normal conscious state, feeling rested and relaxed.

People have approached me with amusing, even ludicrous demands. A few years after I started practicing hypnotherapy, an elderly gentleman came with an unusual request. He said 'Doctor, I am 65, my physical condition is of 55 and my mind is at 45; could you change me to 45?' They think that hypnosis is like a fairy's magic wand that can achieve the impossible or a magic formula that can restore youth like a *"Sanjeevani"* mantra. It is true that a person can remain active mentally and physically and ward off many health problems by using the power of mind. This is evident from the lives of the great Sages and Yogic Masters. But that needs constant effort on the part of the person in the form of self-discipline and regular practice of mind control. Hypnotherapy can help in it, but not a short cut to it.

What one should understand is that hypnosis is not magic or a miracle formula, but a tool that allows the person to go into the inner recesses of his/her mind, bring out the conflicting/disturbing associations and clear them from there, which leads to catharsis and healing. Here the person's mind is working to effect the change and the therapist is acting as a facilitator. So, hypnotherapy will be successful only when the person being hypnotised is willing; it cannot be forced upon the person. Hypnotherapy is used to cater to the needs of the client and not to satisfy the family or others in his/her life. So, a therapist has to respect the client's feelings and not to yield to other's demands. It is also not possible to make the person say or do something which is against his/her strong convictions, because every individual has his/her 'free will' that they can use.

I am pointing this out specifically because I get demands from the parents/spouse/children like 'doctor, please put this idea into his mind.' Or in some cases where the husband/wife suspects of infidelity of spouse, comes to get evidence to verify his/her suspicions by making the person confess under hypnosis. In an extreme case, a man brought his wife and demanded that I hypnotise the wife and the husband will ask questions to her. When I said it is not possible, he got furious and stamped out of my office taking his wife with him. This is all because of the wrong concepts and misinformation that people have about hypnotherapy. Hypnotherapy uses hypnosis for the good of the client, and through that the good of humanity and hypnosis is done with the consent and willingness of the person. If done against his/her wish, it may not succeed.

A clear understanding of hypnotherapy and how it works will show that it is a very safe and effective method of treatment, provided it is done by a qualified person. The purpose of this book is to present hypnosis and hypnotherapy in the right perspective and in a simple way so that people can understand its therapeutic value and benefit from it.

Chapter Two

Power of the Subconscious Mind

The modern medicine man has gained so much power over certain diseases through drugs that he has forgotten about the potential strength within the patient.

– Bernie Siegel

After spending more than three decades in scientific research, a significant part of it on brain development and behavior, when I was doing the course in Clinical hypnotherapy, I found the study of mind intriguing. I had to learn much and revamp my learning and concept about the mind. The Indian Rishis and Sages of old have been searching into the depths of the phenomenon called mind for millennia and have given many insights into it. Still not even a fraction of it is revealed to the common man and studies are still going on in India and abroad. *"Chitta"* is the Sanskrit word used in the ancient Indian scripts to describe mind; but as we are aware, there is no exact equivalent of the word *"Chitta"* in English, neither is there any equivalent to the English word 'mind' in the Indian languages. As already mentioned in the previous chapter, mind is the biggest mystery. As I read more and more about it, from my scientific perspective I found it a challenging study. Different people identify mind with the brain, the third eye or *"Aajna"* chakra, or even the heart. But it remains an abstract concept which cannot be seen or identified with any organ or physical structure. Here I would like to give a basic idea of mind, as used in hypnotherapy, which may help the reader to better understand the further chapters.

The adult human mind is conceived of in two parts: the conscious mind and subconscious mind, which could be considered the rough equivalents to the Sanskrit words *"Manas"* and *"Chitta"* respectively, used in the ancient Indian scripts. All animals, including the humans, are born with the subconscious mind, which is the instinctual part. Conscious mind is a later addition developed a few years after birth in humans, but animals do not seem to develop it.

Conscious mind is the thinking, logical, analyzing part, and functions in relative time and has a short memory. Therefore, we may not be able to recollect something that happened during the early childhood or infancy. It occupies about 12% of the total mind. During our waking hours, the conscious mind is in control of our actions, which at the physical level is executed by the brain.

Subconscious mind is the instinctive, impulsive, and intuitive part. It constitutes about 88% of the total mind and is 8 to 9 times more powerful than the conscious mind. Hypnotherapy works at the subconscious level, while psychology addresses the conscious mind. The basic instinct of any living thing is that of survival or self-preservation, which is the area of subconscious mind. It works on the 'pleasure-pain' principle. What is known, i.e. anything that has been experienced, identified and associated before, and, therefore, does not represent any threat, is accepted as pleasure; and unknowns, i.e. not experienced before and carries no identification or association, and, therefore, perceived as threatening, are pain for the subconscious mind. It keeps a record of everything that happens in our life, identified as pain and pleasure, stored in its memory that cannot be erased. During sleep and during hypnosis the subconscious mind is in charge and its action at the physical level is controlled by the autonomic nervous system, which is formed of the sympathetic and parasympathetic systems.

Subconscious mind does not differentiate between reality and imagination/fantasy; everything is real to it and accepted without asking questions. It does not have any concept of time or space and everything happens as of 'now'; once accepted it gets stored as the reality. You must have observed small children telling exaggerated stories of what they have seen or imagined or heard, like a ghost of gigantic size touching the sky or a huge snake with its hood the size of a big umbrella, etc. The adults laugh at them without realizing that when the child describes so, it is actually seeing it that way; because the child lives in the subconscious, whatever it imagines becomes its reality. This property of the subconscious mind is made use of in hypnotherapy.

There are two types of memory: **modern memory** and **primitive memory**. Modern memory has a record of everything that happens after taking birth in the present body, from the mother's womb to the current moment. It is possible to re-write it if the person wants, and help in changing attitudes, behavior etc. Primitive memory comes from the experiences of the previous births or past lives, brought with the soul when it enters the body of the fetus. Subconscious mind can access any memory of any event in our life/lives, irrespective of its occurrence in relative time.

Subconscious mind reacts through the fight-flight mechanism, either confront and fight back aggressively or take flight and escape from the situation, as seen in animals when they face a threatening situation. Playing dead is the extreme kind of flight reaction in animals. Depression can be considered to be its equivalent in modern man.

When a child is born it has only the subconscious mind. It does not have the ability to think, analyze, reason out or deliberate on its actions. It functions on instinct and impulses, and it does not have any inhibitions. That is why a child blurts out whatever it feels without thinking how others will take it. From the time of birth the child gets exposed to the outside world and starts picking up messages from the surroundings, in verbal and non-verbal (gestures, tone, facial expression, etc.) forms, which the mind identifies as pleasure or pain, and stores in the modern memory. A child learns by identification and association, e.g. when the child feels hungry it gets milk (food) from the mother, so it identifies feeling of hunger with milk and associates it with mother. It is believed that a child of about 18 months, even if it cannot speak, has a vocabulary of about 15000 words stored in its memory. A newborn child has only two fears, fear of falling and fear of loud noise. All other fears are learned and can be unlearned.

By 8 years of age the child's mind builds a library of information that forms a life script for its future reference. This is different from the script brought by the soul, and it dictates the attitudes and habits the person develops. It is influenced by the people, the do's and don'ts dictated by the parents and elders and the environment in which the child grows up.

The conscious mind develops from 8 years to about 13 years of age. Thus, the subconscious is the basic mind and conscious mind is a later addition. In a child the information is stored in its full strength, as there is no filtering by the conscious mind. Therefore, childhood traumas could have a higher impact on the person's later behavior. Many problems in the adult might have their origin in the childhood.

Mind receives information through four different sources: the environment (through the sense organs), the physical body (the sensations and feelings), the conscious mind, and the subconscious mind. Out of these the subconscious mind is the most influential.

The information first reaches the conscious mind in the form of message units (MU) and remains there till the person sleeps. The conscious mind analyses it, referring to the rules and norms of the family, society, culture, teachings, etc. and feedback from the subconscious mind on previous similar experiences stored in the modern memory, then a decision is taken as to the action needed in that situation. The subconscious mind plays a decisive role in the decision making. This decision is conveyed to the brain, which sends signals to the body cells for the required action, synchronizes and coordinates it. Thus, the command comes from the mind and the brain executes it.

Power of Subconscious Mind

Once the person sleeps all the information received by the conscious mind during the day, with its interpretations and conclusions, are transferred to the subconscious mind. The subconscious mind sorts them out, identifies as pleasure or pain, and stores the relevant ones in the modern memory. Once accepted and stored it becomes the reality for the mind and can affect his/her later behavior. If too many message units (information) accumulate in the conscious mind, the person may become tired and go to sleep and the information passes on to the subconscious mind without getting analyzed. The strength of any information depends on how quickly it reaches the modern memory. The longer the information remains in the conscious mind the weaker it becomes, as its strength deteriorates with time. So, the information received immediately before going to sleep is stored in memory in full strength. That is why the last thing you study before going to sleep is more easily recalled than those studied earlier in the day. Many of you must have experienced it, at least when you were preparing for the exams. The information goes to the subconscious mind and gets stored only after the person goes to sleep. So, it is necessary to have a relaxed sleep in the night. Students who study the whole night sacrificing their sleep may have problem in recalling what they studied when they need it during the exams.

Unwanted and surplus message units are discarded through dreams. There are three types of dreams: processing dreams, predictive dreams, and venting dreams. Throwing out of discarded message units is done through the venting dreams. These are the dreams that occur during the last part of our sleep period and which we wake up with.

As already mentioned, the subconscious mind is at a level where time and space are not recognized, and fantasy and fact are not differentiated. So, whatever it imagines or visualizes becomes a fact and accepted as the reality. It can even make things happen by imagining them. This property of the subconscious mind is made use of in bringing about positive changes in feelings, attitudes, behavior and in health. For example, when a person comes to a hypnotherapist for help in improving public speaking skill, the therapist makes him/her imagine or visualize, under hypnosis, each detail of the performance in front of the audience, recreating the whole scenario from the start to finish, which the mind accepts as the reality and stores in the modern memory and becomes the known. When the person actually goes to speak, that memory guides him at every step. This can also be done by the person himself/herself under self-hypnosis (discussed later in this book).

Habit Formation

An experience or thought stimulates the secretion of electro-chemicals in the brain. Neuropathways are created and the chemicals flow through these pathways, carrying the signals. Every time an experience is repeated the chemicals take the same pathway and the pathway gets reinforced and strengthened. For example, when a person smokes for the first time that experience generates a thought and stimulates the secretion of the electrochemical and a pathway is created. Subconscious mind stores the memory. When he smokes again the chemical takes the same pathway and the subconscious mind identifies the feeling as pleasure because it is known and adds to the memory. Every time the person smokes it reinforces the neuropathway and the feeling gets strengthened, and it becomes a habit. Once strongly established, it becomes difficult for the person to break out of the habit, as in the case of smoking, because it becomes the comfort zone for the mind, a known and, therefore, a pleasurable experience. When the person wants to change it consciously, conflict develops between the conscious and subconscious minds, because the subconscious mind views the change, in this case not smoking, as pain as it is unknown to it and rejects it. Such habits can be broken, and more positive alternatives can be installed through suggestions under hypnosis, if the person is willing and committed to change. The therapist helps the client to convert the unknown into known, therefore, accept it as pleasure and a new neuropathway is created. This is reinforced by repeating the suggestion in subsequent sessions, strengthening this neuropathway and establishing the changed feeling. Thus, even firmly established habits can be changed with the help of hypnotherapy if the person desires it strongly and works sincerely for it.

Chapter Three

Hypnosis and Hypnotherapy

All hypnosis is self-hypnosis. The hypnotherapist is a facilitator.

– A. M. Krasner (Founder, American Institute of Hypnotherapy)

'I am driving on a familiar road, there is not much traffic. I am relaxed and driving leisurely. A melodious song from an old Hindi film is playing on the stereo, which is one of my favorites. My memories go back to the College days, when I had watched the movie with my best friend and hostel mate. I am so engrossed in my thoughts that I miss the turning I have to take and drive ahead. Then I see the petrol pump on my left and suddenly wake up to the present and realise my mistake.' During that short time, I was in hypnosis.

Hypnosis is a trance state in which the person becomes less aware of the surroundings and more acutely focused inwards. It is a state of deep concentration. Each one of us experiences this state several times a day, even though unknown to us; as one is engrossed in an interesting book, listening to music, watching a favorite TV program, deep in thought, daydreaming, etc. When someone touches you or calls out your name, you suddenly wake up with a jerk and become aware of the surroundings. I remember one of my experiences when I was working for my doctorate. I was deeply engrossed in my experiment that I did not know when my Professor came and stood near me. A chuckle from my fellow student brought me back to reality and I noticed the Professor watching me with an amused look. All of you will have many such experiences to recount. It is a natural phenomenon, but its occurrence and duration are not under our control. Hypnosis can be induced under controlled conditions and can be used for resolving behavioral issues, emotional problems and treating diseases. Treatment using hypnosis is called '**hypnotherapy**.'

Hypnotherapy, as known today, is rather a young branch of healing disciplines. A brief account of its evolution will be interesting to the readers.

History of Hypnotherapy

Hypnosis has been known to humanity for millennia, although not in that name. Use of hypnosis in healing was prevalent in many ancient civilizations in India, Egypt, and Greece, with a known history of more than 5000 years. Shamans or tribal medicine men of Asia, Africa and America are known to take their patients into a trance state as a part of the healing process. In Greece, a healing room called the 'sleep chamber' was used; treatment was done by building expectation and creating a trance state by repeated chanting in a soothing environment. Meditation, a form of self-hypnosis, has been a part of ancient Hindu culture and a way of life, but was known only in India. It was Swami Vivekananda who introduced it in 1893 to the outside world.

In modern medical history the first use of hypnosis is claimed to be by Dr. Franz Anton Mesmer (1733–1815), a physician from Vienna, Austria, in the 18th century. He believed that many objects contained a magnetic fluid with healing power that can be transferred to the patients for cure. He called it 'animal magnetism.' He shifted to France, where he treated thousands of patients using this method, came to be known as "Mesmerism" (from Mesmer). The Marquis de Puysegur, a student of Mesmer, did research on this healing energy and concluded that it is not magnetic, but electrical and is present in all living things, including plants. He found that the patients went to sleep, but they could talk. He called it 'artificial somnambulism.' Abbe Faria (1756–1819), a catholic monk, was born (there is some controversy on his date of birth) in Portuguese Goa in India, but lived and practiced mesmerism in Europe; he called it 'lucid sleep.' He is considered to be the first person to approach hypnosis and clairvoyance as a science. He rejected the animal magnetism concept of Mesmer and stated that hypnosis worked by the power of suggestion. He was later patronized by the French emperor Napoleon Bonaparte, and it is said that the emperor consulted him before the battles he fought.

Mesmerism was practiced by several medical doctors in England and some European countries like France, Spain and Germany. Many of them found that although the patients appeared to be sleeping, they were able to hear the mesmerist and respond to him. Dr. James Braid, a Scottish Surgeon, got interested in mesmerism after seeing it in a travelling show. He called this sleep-like state the 'nervous sleep' and gave the name hypnosis in 1843 (after "Hypnos," the Greek God of sleep) to describe this condition. He was the first to introduce it to the English-speaking world. It gained popularity in the 19th century. In the second half of the 19th century, Ambroise-Auguste Liebeault and Hippolyte Bernheim in Nancy, France, started the Nancy School program of hypnosis. The Nancy school opened the subject to a new generation of medical students who started research on mesmerism. Liebeault called it "suggestive therapeutics." Emile Coue, a French psychologist got interested in suggestive therapeutics. He was the earliest proponent of self-hypnosis and auto-suggestion. Sigmund Freud, the world renowned Psychotherapist, used hypnotherapy in the early days of his practice, but later discarded it and changed to psychoanalysis and association for behavioral therapy.

Hypnotherapy declined in popularity during the early part of the last century but got revived in the 1950s. Clark Hull (1884–1952), a Psychologist and behavioral scientist, did extensive investigations on hypnosis and conducted seminars at the University of Wisconsin, USA. One of his students, Milton Erickson (1901–1980), got fascinated by a demo and started experimenting on it. He developed a number of methods for hypnosis induction which are used in modern hypnotherapy. Erickson and John Kappas (1925–2002), founder of the Hypnosis Motivation Institute, USA, contributed significantly to the development of hypnotherapy to the present status. Some Army hospitals used hypnosis on soldiers returning from World War II, suffering from trauma, fear and dissociation. Hypnotherapy was recognised by the British Medical Association (1955) and the American Medical Association (1958). Currently it is being used in several countries not only for treating psychological issues but also many physical diseases.

What is Hypnosis?

Hypnosis is a state of altered level of awareness, also considered to be the fourth state of consciousness, different from the other states of waking, dreaming and sleep. However, this is different from the fourth state described in the Upanishads of India; Mandukya Upanishad describes the fourth state as *"Turya,"* which is a much higher state of meditation, which is pure consciousness, where the person rises above all mental awareness, beyond time and space, transcends the subject-object duality, and all thoughts and even experience of nothingness disappear. Even though hypnosis is much deeper than waking and dreaming states, where the distinction between past, present and future disappears and everything is seen as now, it cannot be identified with the *"Turya"* state. In hypnosis the mind awareness is still there at the conscious level, but deep buried memories, not available in the conscious waking state, can be accessed in this state.

Hypnosis is characterized by deep relaxation, focused attention, acute sensory perception and hyper-suggestibility (increased receptivity to suggestions). Other features include shallow breathing, flaccid facial muscles, inability to voluntary movements, sometimes slurring of speech and flowing of tears. Even though the person appears to be sleeping, the condition is different from that experienced during the normal sleep state. During the waking state, the conscious mind is awake and in control, and the subconscious mind, though awake, does not have control. During natural sleep, the conscious mind goes to sleep, and the person remains unconscious of the surroundings, the sounds and activities around; therefore, new learning is not possible in this condition. Under hypnosis the conscious mind remains awake, even though the subconscious mind is in control, and learning is possible in this state. This property is made use of in hypnotherapy.

In hypnosis, the level of trance can be light, medium or deep, classified as depths. Depth is a concept to know the most receptive state of mind when to give suggestions that are accepted easily without resistance. Conscious mind, as a fact, feels a need to analyze and reason out every information it receives. Under hypnosis this process is disorganised so that message units (information received) are passed on to the subconscious mind without being analyzed or filtered. According to John Kappas, conscious mind can handle a maximum of 4000 message units (MUs) per minute. Increasing the MUs above this will lead to anxiety and loss of control of the conscious mind. Overloading the conscious mind with message units to a high level, above its capacity to handle them, makes it confused and it reverts back to the primitive instinct of fight-flight response, handing over control to the subconscious mind, resulting in hypnosis. The loss of control by the conscious mind is a gradual process, without it actually realizing that it is losing control, starting from the shallow state, the light trance where the conscious mind retains some control, to the very deep state, where the subconscious mind is totally in charge and the person becomes highly receptive to verbal suggestions. Hypnotherapy uses hypnosis to enhance the receptivity to the therapist's suggestion, so that the suggestion goes directly into the subconscious mind without getting analyzed by the conscious mind and becomes accepted.

Even light trance gives good relaxation to the mind and body, which gives benefit to a person under stress, as seen from the following example.

> I was on a flight from Bhopal to Mumbai. The journey lasts about 2 and half hours. I was in the window seat. A young couple occupied the other two seats, the lady sitting next to me with her husband in the aisle seat. As the aircraft started moving, she started vomiting and by the time the flight took off she had filled 3 air sickness bags with her vomit, still the vomiting continuing. I gently placed my palm on her hand and said softly 'just recline, close your eyes and relax' and she leaned back and closed her eyes. With my palm still on her hand, I whispered 'relax' several times and she became relaxed and the vomiting stopped. Then I gave a suggestion, speaking almost in a whisper 'you are relaxed; now sleep comfortably till we reach Mumbai. The moment the flight lands in Mumbai you will wake up, fully rested and refreshed.' She slept peacefully throughout the journey and the moment we landed in Mumbai she opened her eyes with a smile and no evidence of discomfort.

Since she was under a lot of anxiety, she was already in a semi-hypnotic state; so it was easy to take her into hypnosis by simply relaxing her further and she became receptive to my suggestion and benefited from it, even though it was a light trance.

Generally, three depths are recognized: hypnoidal, cataleptic, and somnambulistic. Hypnoidal stage is light trance or the alpha state, characterized by deep relaxation, shallow and rhythmic breathing and rapid eye movement. Self-hypnosis can take one to this state. It can be achieved by meditation also. Suggestions for self-improvement and changing some attitudes, repeated in several consecutive sessions are effective in this state.

Cataleptic stage is medium trance state. It is characterized by deeper relaxation, sometimes lacrimation (tears rolling down) and slower speech. Suggestions for changing certain habits and attitudes, building confidence, self-esteem, improving study habits, etc. given in this stage are found to be effective.

Somnambulistic stage is the deepest of the three stages, the theta state, in which relaxation is even deeper; flushing of face, lacrimation, slurring of speech and partial or total amnesia can occur. There is no interference from the conscious mind and suggestions are easily accepted without resistance and implemented by the subconscious mind. Therefore, this stage is used for therapeutic purposes.

Time distortion is possible under hypnosis; a session lasting one hour may seem 10 minutes or less, a 10 minutes session may seem one hour or more. Many people think that they did not go into hypnosis, as they could hear everything I said. As I mentioned earlier, the conscious mind is awake and listening, that is why hypnotherapy works. One of my clients on waking up after an one hour session said that he did not go into hypnosis, then he looked at the clock and exclaimed 'oh it is one hour, then I must have been in hypnosis.' He was under the impression that he had been on the couch for about 10 minutes.

Hypnotherapy uses the power of the subconscious mind for bringing about changes at the emotional, mental and physical planes that result in better understanding of oneself and others, resolve internal conflicts, clear mental distortions and cure functional and physical disorders. This is done without the help of any medicines, purely through suggestions. In this respect, it is similar to psychotherapy, but differs from the latter in that while psychotherapy addresses the conscious mind, which is only about 12% of the total mind, hypnotherapy works with the subconscious mind, which is about 88% of the total mind and is 8–9 times more powerful than the conscious mind. In most emotional problems, hypnotherapy produces faster and more permanent effects, achieving similar or better results in 2–3 sessions compared to 10–15 sessions of psychotherapy. As the suggestions go directly to the subconscious mind, the seat of stored memory, the client can access the disturbing emotions and release them from there, removing the problem from the root.

Chapter Four

Pre-Induction Interview, its Purpose and Advantages

When a prospective client approaches me seeking help in resolving some issue, as the therapist, it is my endeavor to know the details about the person, the problem and its course of development, his/her medical history, etc. This is achieved by a face to face talk with the person and asking proper questions that help him/her to provide the required information. In terms of hypnotherapy, this process is known as the 'pre-induction interview.' Before taking into hypnosis, I, as any other hypnotherapist, do a thorough interview of the person, and, if needed, question other members of the family also. This is the opportunity to get to know the client and his/her background and gather detailed information about the problem and its development and make him/her ready for hypnosis. I can get the required information only if the client feels free to open up in front of me and prepared to share all that he/she knows about the problem and answer my queries truthfully. This is possible only if the client trusts me as the person who will help him/her in achieving the goals and in whom he/she can confide without any inhibition. Therefore, apart from gathering information about the problem, a main purpose of the interview is to build rapport with the client and make him/her feel comfortable with the therapist. The client is encouraged to speak freely, express his/her feelings and clarify doubts and apprehensions.

One question most clients ask me, when we start the interview, is that if I will share the information with the family/spouse or others. I assure the client that whatever is revealed in the room will be kept confidential. As a policy of confidentiality, when an adult client is interviewed or hypnotised, I do not allow anyone else to sit there unless the client wants it, except in the case of patients of major depression, who may not be able to respond properly. I also do not reveal any details of the interview without permission of the client. Even when a case is discussed in a meeting or in an article, the identity of the person is kept hidden. With children it is different; at least one parent or guardian who accompanies the child is asked to be present.

A person coming for hypnotherapy may have undergone other types of treatment without getting much benefit and this may be his/her last resort and hope. They may come with a lot of expectations, sometimes even unrealistic. In my experience, the first question many people ask when they call me for an appointment, even before telling the problem, is if they can be cured in one session. These are people who have been trying other treatments for several years but are not satisfied with the results. But they expect a miracle cure from hypnotherapy. Here I would like to mention that we in hypnotherapy do not generally use the word 'cure' as it implies a disease. A hypnotherapist handles many issues which are not considered a medical problem or disease. Moreover, in hypnotherapy the treatment outcome is decided, to a great extent, by the client, because if the person is not prepared for the change the therapist cannot do much. The therapist only helps the persons to help themselves in achieving the desired result. So before starting the treatment, it is necessary to understand the actual problem that the person is facing at the emotional, mental and physical levels, what are his/her expectations and what he/she wants to achieve from the therapy. Unlike in the conventional treatments, hypnotherapists do not have any method to objectively assess the condition that can help in diagnosing the problem. The only tool is questioning the person in detail to extract the required information. This is done during the pre-induction interview by asking the person directly, or in case of small children talking to the parents, siblings, etc. I explain these to the client so that he/she understands the importance of his/her willing participation and total involvement in the healing process.

One has to develop a skill to ask the right questions in the right manner, so that the client opens up and talks without inhibition and answers the questions truthfully. Therefore, building rapport with the client is the first step, so that the client feels confident about you as the therapist and as the person whom he/she can trust and build expectation. Unlike in USA, UK and some European countries, where hypnotherapy is accepted in several hospitals as a complementary and alternative therapy along with modern medical treatments, e.g. Mayo Clinic, USC School of Dentistry, USA, etc., it is not commonly practiced as a routine in the hospitals in India. Most of the clients do not have any idea about it but may have apprehensions and fears originating from what they gather from stage shows, television and other visual media. Therefore, they may be afraid of hypnosis, and may have many doubts to be clarified. It is necessary to remove their fears and make them comfortable with the therapist and hypnosis. A purpose of the pre-induction interview is to clarify the client's doubts and dispel fears, so that they can accept hypnotherapy as a safe method of treatment and become ready for it. Therefore, during the interview they are encouraged to ask questions and get their doubts clarified.

Hypnotherapy is a partnership between the therapist and the client; the actual healing is done by the client, while the therapist functions as a facilitator, providing the guidance and opportunity to bring about the change. This is possible only if the client is willing to cooperate and go along with the therapist. Therefore, some of the main purposes of the interview is to build rapport and remove the fears and apprehensions that make the client hesitant to accept hypnotherapy and also build hope and expectation in the client. This is the responsibility of the therapist and pre-induction interview provides the platform for it. When I explain hypnosis and what the client can expect from hypnotherapy it helps create credibility and trust and prepares the person for the session. Detailed information about the client's disturbing issues is gathered during the interview.

Gathering Information

Most of the time, the problem first given by the clients when they come may not be the real one. The person may tell you the medical diagnosis received from the earlier consultations in hospitals, based on the physical symptoms and clinical tests, or what they think, based on information gained from others or literature or internet. A 13 year old boy told me that he has schizophrenia, although he did not know what it means. He had heard the word from the doctor when the latter was discussing the child's problem with his parents. As a hypnotherapist I do not go by the physical or physiological symptoms only, but look for the emotional feelings that trigger the symptoms, i.e. the subconscious factors that are at the root of the problem, and bring out the real issue by asking probing questions.

> A lady in her early 40s came to me with the complaint that she is not able to concentrate. When asked if she has any other problems, she repeatedly said that there is nothing else and that if she can concentrate everything will be fine. Further questioning revealed that she is under a lot of stress and is not able to relax and her sleep is disturbed. I explained that relaxation is a pre-requisite for concentration, and we will start with that and she agreed. So, the first two sessions were used for de-stressing and relaxation, followed by another session in which suggestion to build confidence was given and her problem with concentration was resolved.

Sometimes the medical diagnosis can bias a client towards imagining symptoms that are not actually there. A 52 year old man came to me with the diagnosis of depression for which he was taking medicines for the last 6 or 7 years. When I asked him about his symptoms and feelings, he gave me a page from a popular health magazine and said these are his symptoms. It was an article on depression that gave a general description of the disease and listed about 15 symptoms. As he was clinically diagnosed with depression, after reading the article he started imagining each one of the symptoms applicable to him. But the fact is that if he had all those symptoms, he would not have been able to come by himself and travel alone as he had done that day.

Therefore, gathering information about the actual problem is an essential part of pre-induction interview, as also to find out the client's expectations and what they want to achieve from this therapy. This is done by asking probing questions into the problem and its course of development, the treatments he/she has taken, and the benefits obtained and what prompted the client to think of hypnotherapy and consulting me. However, we have to be careful not to create negative impression in the client's mind or ask leading questions that can influence his/her response. While forming the questions I try to follow some guidelines that have helped me in getting the relevant information without unnecessarily prolonging the interview. As far as possible, I keep my questions strictly connected to the problem and avoid irrelevant topics, unless there are indications to turn to topics that may have a seeming relation to or influence on the development of the problem. Sometimes a client may stray from the main subject, then I have to intervene and redirect him/her back to the relevant issue, gently and in an inoffensive manner. It is the client who has to probe into his/her mind for the answers. So, it is wise to avoid leading questions that can give clues on which he/she can build up. So, I try my best to keep the questions open, so that the client has to find the answers from his/her own experiences. If the client is not able to tell in the cognitive state, questions can be asked under hypnosis and the right answers will come from the subconscious mind.

For proper therapy, the therapist must know the specifics of a problem, not generalizations. So, when the client states the problem in a generalized way, I always make it a point to get the specifics by probing deeper through further questions. For example, one of my clients stated his problem as 'no mind control.' When I asked him what he would like to achieve from the therapy, he simply said 'I want peace of mind.' These are very generalized statements and do not give any information about his real issue. I had to ask several questions, gradually probing deeper and deeper into the issue and after about 10 minutes of questioning he started providing more details. He was living in a joint family, including his parents and grandparents, father's two brothers and their families. Compared to his cousins, he was not doing well financially, and this invited criticisms, and he was under a lot of stress. He was feeling depressed and suffered from inferiority feeling. He had been to other counsellors and to a couple of psychiatrists and taken medicines without getting any lasting benefit. In the course of these processes he had forgotten what his actual problem was. While looking for the answers to my questions, he started seeing the problem with more clarity and from an emotional perspective. Open-ended questions prompt the client to search deep into his/her mind for the answer, analyze and reorganize it, and get to the specifics of the problem. Once I came to know the specifics of the problem, it was possible to plan the treatment, which was successfully completed.

Many people are reluctant to tell their real problem due to fear of what others will think. The clients often request me not to tell anybody, especially the family members and relatives, that they have consulted me. Some parents also try to hide details. When a young lady, a professional degree student, experiencing fear and severe anxiety was brought to me,

I asked her mother if she knows of any traumatic event the client may have gone through as a child. She said there is nothing she knows of and her daughter had a happy and secure childhood. Sometimes we have to ask the parents about childhood incidences as the client may not remember them, even though such incidences can impact his/her later behavior. In this case there were clues to indicate such a possibility, even though the client did not remember. But under hypnosis she told about sexual abuse by a friend of her father when she was 6 or 7 years. After the session again I asked the mother if she knows about it. Then she said that she knew it but did not think it important as her daughter is now an adult.

We are trying to help the clients to achieve what they want and create the feeling that they expect to experience when they achieve it. Therefore, during the interview it is important to find out their expectation from the therapy, what they desire to achieve and how will they feel on achieving it. These are the motivations that brought them for therapy and can be included in the suggestion. I always make it a point to note down everything in the client's own words and use as many of them as possible in the suggestion. Since they are their words, they will be easily accepted by their mind when given as a suggestion under hypnosis.

Every type of therapy has its own merits and de-merits. So, I feel that when discussing the client's experience with the other treatment modalities we must refrain from comparing or criticising them. If the client has opted for a therapy, he/she has a reason for it, and we must accept that. But when they come to me, I try to do my best that I can to realise their reasonable expectations and justify their trust in me as a hypnotherapist.

Once the real problem is unearthed, suggestion can be framed and given to the client under hypnosis. This is explained in the next chapter.

Chapter Five
Hypnotherapy Session and Post Hypnotic Suggestions

Once the required information about the client and his/her problem is obtained, we are now ready for the actual therapy. A typical hypnotherapy session includes 3 main steps and lasts from 60 to 75 minutes. The first session can take longer, as the pre-induction interview, as described in the previous chapter, is done in that session.

The 3 main steps are:

1. Induction of hypnosis.
2. Post-hypnotic suggestions and other therapeutic interventions.
3. Bringing out of hypnosis.

Induction of Hypnosis

Before inducing hypnosis, I do a quick test to know the hypnotisability of the client. The same method may not work for all types of people, because people differ in the level of their hypnotisability, in the hypnotherapist's terms, suggestibility of the person. Some are more suggestible and easier to hypnotise, while some others are more resistant. In my experience most people can be hypnotised by using the right method; there are only 2–3 percent of people who are really difficult to hypnotise, because they are highly analytical and have a fear of being controlled by the hypnotist.

As mentioned in chapter 3, hypnosis is induced by overloading the mind with message units, disorganizing the analytical capacity of the conscious mind, so that it is unable to handle the information and hands over control to the subconscious mind. Currently several methods are available for hypnotic induction, from the elaborate hand levitation to the very short induction by handshake or shock induction. Many free scripts are available on the net. The most common methods use verbal suggestions, the hypnotist repeatedly suggesting to the client that he/she is entering a trance state, feeling relaxed and calm, gradually leading into that state. Non-verbal methods use devises like pendulum, hypno-disk, crystal ball, etc. My preferred methods are those using verbal suggestions. But it may not be possible to use them in small children or people with some disabilities, where pendulum or other devices are used. In children between 5 and 10 years I have found story telling very effective, because they live most of the time in a fantasy world and it is easy for them to relate to fictional characters.

In most cases, the depth reached by the initial induction may not be enough for therapy. In the first induction most people go to the hypnoidal stage, some may reach the cataleptic stage. More depths are achieved through further suggestions.

Post-Hypnotic Suggestions

Suggestions given after the client is in hypnosis are called post-hypnotic suggestions. They include deepening suggestions, suggestions to resolve the client's issues and suggestion to bring out of hypnosis.

Deepening suggestions are given to increase the depth of hypnosis, taking the client farther and farther away from control of the conscious mind and deeper and deeper into the subconscious mind; deep somnambulistic stage is preferred for most treatments, although simple suggestions for improving study habits in children work well in the cataleptic stage also. I use several methods to take the client into a very deep somnambulistic stage before treating emotional and physical problems. In some cases, I have found that the client sometimes revert back to a shallower state. But if they are in a very deep state, even if they come up they still remain in a highly suggestible state so that the therapy is not interrupted; otherwise they can be taken to the required depth by giving further suggestions. The purpose is to completely remove any influence of the conscious mind and reach the most receptive state of mind so that the client will accept the suggestion for change without resistance.

Both induction and deepening are important in hypnotherapy. As in the case of induction, deepening is also done through verbal suggestions. Progressive relaxation, visualizing or imagining each part of the body, from head to feet or from feet to head, becoming relaxed, is a good method of deepening. This method can be used also for induction.

Suggestions to Resolve the Client's Issues

This is the actual treatment. These are suggestions for bringing about the desired changes and help in resolving the disturbing issues. They include suggestions to change negative attitudes, stop undesirable behavioral patterns or habits, to improve performance skills, stopping addictive habits like smoking, drinking etc., resolve inter-personal conflicts, or for treating emotional problems, in effect to bring about the changes that the client desires to achieve.

While framing the suggestions I try my best to include the client's words, especially what he/she desires to achieve, their expectations from the therapy, and the feelings they would like to get once they achieve what they want, to make the suggestion more apt in addressing his/her specific problem; it can be said to be person- and problem-oriented. Except for general stress reduction, confidence building, etc. where common suggestions work, I write down separate suggestion for each client and, where possible and if desired, get his/her approval before hypnotising the person.

In framing the suggestions, I follow some general guidelines, as listed below, as far as possible.

1. Using a positive language, e.g. in a suggestion for removing fear, I say *"you are feeling confident/bold/courageous"* instead of *"you are not afraid"* or *"you are not feeling scared."* In the suggestion to quit smoking, it will be *"you are a non-smoker"* instead of *"you do not smoke."*

2. Using motivating statements. Power words, even exaggerations are used for emphasis sometimes, which will be accepted by the subconscious mind; e. g. excellent, wonderful, marvelous, on top of the world, etc.

3. Using the present or present continuous tense because the subconscious mind does not recognize time. It functions always in the present, e.g. suggestion for confidence building will be *"you feel confident"* or *"you are feeling confident"* instead of *"you will feel confident."* I sometimes use future tense in situations where a delayed action is indicated, e.g. preparing for an interview scheduled for a later date.

4. Using sentences suggesting that the desired change has already occurred; e.g. for a person facing a job interview, making it sound as if the person is already achieving the goal, like answering all the questions correctly, speaking confidently, and getting selected; ending on a positive note, like *'feeling very happy and going home with a smile of satisfaction.'* This has been found to be very successful in achieving the desired effect.

5. In one session I repeat the suggestion 3 times; this is done to reinforce the suggestion, so that it will be better accepted and more firmly instilled in the subconscious memory. We have to remember that when we change an established pattern of thought or behavior, what we are doing is changing a known and replacing it with an unknown and make the mind accept it as pleasure. So, we are trying to overcome the resistance towards the unknown and make it acceptable as the new known, which is pleasurable. The more a message is repeated, the more real it becomes to the subconscious mind and accepted as the truth.

6. I frame the suggestion for one issue at a time, taking care not to club different issues together, as it can create confusion. So, if a person lists many issues, I ask him/her to arrange them in the order of priority and address each one in that order in further sessions.

Other Therapeutic Interventions

In treating issues like fears, phobias, anxiety, interpersonal conflicts, physical diseases, addictive habits, etc. simple suggestions alone may not be enough to completely eliminate the problem. In such cases we use additional methods like desensitization, positive visualization, guided imagery, hypnodrama, etc.

In **desensitization** we take the client into a deep somnambulistic stage and in that state ask the client to go to a situation in which he/she experiences the feeling. Once the person imagines the situation, he/she is asked to bring up the feeling and release it, and then fill the vacant space with a positive feeling. The release is done gradually in a step-by-step manner in 3–5 rounds in one session, till the person feels comfortable in the situation. Then the replacement feeling is reinforced by verbal suggestion. I do not have to know what feelings the clients bring up and release, as long as their mind is doing it, because the subconscious mind knows what to do.

Even one session has been found to bring about the desired change in some cases. In one of my workshops, even though not a part of the program, I offered to do a demo for the benefit of the participants.

> One of the participants, let us call him Renjit, was talking aggressively and in an irritating way and many participants felt uncomfortable. Renjit volunteered to be the demo subject. I took him into deep hypnosis and asked him to imagine himself in a situation when he felt irritated and aggressive and bring up the feelings experienced in that situation and release it; the process was completed in 3 rounds and filled the space with feeling of calmness; then I woke him up. Immediately after the session we had the tea break and, to the surprise of everyone, he was more cordial and friendly, and his expression was also more pleasant.

I have found desensitization a very effective method in removing fears, phobias, anxiety, sadness, general anger, guilt feeling, etc.

Guided imagery is a method used to improve performance skills like singing, dancing, different kinds of sports, change some habits, etc. in which the person under deep hypnosis is guided through each detail of the process from start to finish, ending up with achieving the desired result. **Hypnodrama** is used to resolve interpersonal issues, acting them out in a safe environment. These are described in more detail in chapter 7.

Bringing out of Hypnosis or Waking the Person Up

As a hypnotherapist, I know that it is essential to bring the person out of hypnosis at the end of the session and make sure that he/she is completely awake and comfortable before allowing him/her to go home. This is very important because under hypnosis the person is in a hyper-suggestible state of mind. If he/she goes out in that state, there are high chances of picking up negative messages from the environment, both verbal and nonverbal, that go directly to the subconscious mind and get stored and become part of the modern memory. This can create false memories and affect the behavior of the person, creating new problems. Therefore, bringing out of hypnosis into the normal waking state is a very important and essential part of any hypnotherapy session. This is done through waking up suggestion and is very fast. I usually count the person up from 1 to 5 and say, 'open your eyes, wide awake,' which works well in all clients. Other methods like snapping fingers or saying the word 'wake' loudly, etc., are being used in practice. Occasionally, on waking up a few clients may feel foggy, heavy or light, a little confused, etc., but say that they are fine. In such cases I put them back to trance, give a short suggestion to relax and then wake the person up. Usually they feel comfortable on waking up.

Sometimes a person may open his/her eyes during the session and wants to go home; but it is not advisable to allow him/her to go in that condition, because the person may still be in a semi-trance. I put the person back to trance and then wake him/her up properly, by giving the waking up suggestion, before allowing him/her to go home. In some cases, the person may slip into natural sleep during the session and do not respond to any suggestion; then I let him/her sleep for about 10 minutes. Usually the person wakes up automatically, otherwise I arouse him/her up.

The first session is the most important. Success of the first session makes further sessions more comfortable for the client and helps in building trust in the therapy and the therapist. Many people have a fear of hypnosis and this will be removed when they experience it. If the first session fails, the therapist can lose the client. A young lady of 26 or 27 years was brought to me by her mother. She had lot of tension and anxiety about her forthcoming marriage. She wanted a counselling but was afraid of hypnosis. I explained her about hypnosis and hypnotherapy and its advantages, giving examples from my experience. Finally, she agreed. She went very deep in a few minutes. In that state I gave suggestion to release the tension, then woke her up. She was very relaxed, felt good and had a smile on her face. She was surprised that hypnosis is so simple; her fear of hypnosis had completely gone. She was eager to do further sessions and fixed the next appointment before she left.

It should be kept in mind that the client's consent is a crucial factor in the success of hypnosis induction and therapy.

Chapter Six
Emotional Basis of Physical Diseases

All I can say as a scientist is that the great majority of physical illnesses have in part some psychosomatic origin.

– Hans Selye

A 38 year old paramedical staff with severe neck pain and stiffness was referred to me. The orthopaedic doctor had diagnosed Spondylitis, prescribed medicines, and advised wearing a cervical collar. He was getting irritated at small things and quarrelled with his colleagues. This was affecting his work, creating a situation that could leave him jobless. He had problems at home also, losing temper at small things and shouting at his wife and son. While talking to him, he revealed that he was under a lot of stress at home. He had to take care of his sick father which he did sincerely. But he felt that his younger brother and his father's brother were telling lies and turning his father against him. He felt angry towards his brother and uncle; their presence bothered him so much that he lost temper at the mere sight of them. But he was not able to express it or prevent them from visiting his father. He started getting severe pain and stiffness in the neck, affecting his profession and even routine activities. After two sessions of hypnotherapy that addressed his stress and anger, the pain and stiffness in the neck reduced significantly and one more session gave complete relief from it and his medicines were stopped. It is one year after hypnotherapy and he is maintaining good health and is happy at home and at workplace and doing well in his profession. This shows how emotions can affect physical health.

Most diseases can be considered as psycho-somatic, i.e. there is a mental/emotional and a physical component to it. As shown in the above case, emotional disturbances can cause physical discomforts. The most common example is the upset stomach that most of us have experienced at some or other time – before going to the exam, job interview, facing an audience, giving a seminar, travelling to a new place, etc. We become so tense and anxious that all our logic and reasoning get topsy-turvy. In such cases releasing the tension and relaxing the person can remove the physical discomfort.

> One of my clients was a 23 year old male student, staying away from home in another state, who was diagnosed with irritable bowel syndrome. Every morning before going to the University he had to go to the toilet several times, and still not satisfied. He tried to avoid travels and going to functions due to the fear that any time he may get the urge to go to toilet, which was embarrassing. He was taking medicines, which did not help much. When he was brought to me by his father, he was very nervous. I relaxed him and explained about hypnotherapy and he agreed. After two sessions to release tension his bowel problem reduced considerably; he was satisfied after going two times to the toilet in the morning. Two more sessions were done to build confidence and self-esteem and his bowel problem disappeared.

Stress is accepted to be behind many health problems; the medical sciences have recognized the role of stress in producing diseases like cancer, diabetes, hypertension and cardiac problems.

Many people are not able to openly express their feelings and, therefore, suppress them. These feelings are internalized and repressed and stored in the modern memory. This is a defence mechanism of the subconscious mind. Sigmund Freud first described repression as the basic defence mechanism of the unconscious mind to save the ego from embarrassment and anxiety. When such emotions are repressed again and again, they get accumulated in the subconscious memory and create emotional blocks that can cause physical symptoms later.

Emotions are energy; there are positive emotions and negative emotions. Positive emotions keep us healthy, while negative emotions create illness. Love is the most positive emotion, the most positive energy. Love and forgiveness can heal all hurts and keep one healthy. Some of the most damaging emotions are grief, fear, anger, hatred, jealousy, and guilt. Holding back and accumulating them blocks the flow of positive energy, leading to sickness. Hypnotherapy helps in releasing the pent-up emotions and clearing the negative energy blocks, leading to catharsis and healing.

Negative emotions like anger, grief, fear, jealousy and guilt can lead to physical problems like cancer, diabetes, cardiac diseases, kidney dysfunction, etc. It can be easily understood if we analyse how emotional disturbances affect the physiology. Stress and negative emotions stimulate the secretion of stress hormones like cortisol which produce free radicals. Free radicals damage cells and cause gene mutations, leading to cell death and diseases. Maintaining a stress free and relaxed state and positive mindset can help in preventing many chronic diseases.

Every person has an aura of about 12 feet around him/her. This consists of the different energy levels or energy bodies; from the lowest, the etheric body immediately enclosing the physical body, through increasing energy levels represented by the astral body, mental body and spiritual body. Physical body and etheric body are the *"Annamaya Kosa"* and *"Praanamaya Kosa,"* respectively, together constituting the 'gross body' described in the Taittiriya Upanishad. Etheric body has the same form as that of the physical body and is destroyed with the latter when the person dies. The other bodies form the subtle bodies and go with the soul, carrying the memories of experiences in that life, which become part of the primitive memory in the next incarnation. The healing energy is the cosmic energy and comes from the Universe to the etheric body through the Chakras. The etheric body distributes it through the *"Nadis"* to every cell of the body. Every Chakra inducts the energy at the frequency specifically required by the tissues, organs and other body parts located near the Chakra points. When there is a block in the energy flow into the chakra systems, it disturbs the smooth flow of cosmic energy to the body parts causing physiological changes, leading to physical diseases.

> A 60 year old housewife, breast cancer survivor, was brought to me by her husband. She was gloomy and depressed. Under deep hypnosis, I asked her to bring up her feelings and release them; she showed anger, as evident in her facial expression and reactions in the right hand and feet. After releasing the feelings, she became relaxed

and calm. On waking up she revealed that she had a long held grudge against her husband. When she delivered her first child, her cousin, a young widow, stayed with them to help her with the baby. Her husband developed a relation with the cousin and neglected his wife and child. But she could not do anything as she needed the help of the cousin. She felt betrayed and angry, but suppressed her feelings, and had strained relationship with her husband. Now they are on better terms and her husband is taking good care of her, but she was not able to forgive him and the hurt remained with her. After the hypnotherapy session she was able to accept her husband and his loving care more fully and benefit from it. Her depression was also cured, and she became more cheerful.

More than 90% of the cancer patients included in a study were found to have a history of long suppressed anger. Other emotions associated with cancers include hatred, jealousy and resentment. Holding back of emotions like grief plays a major role in the development of diabetes.

A 55 year old bank employee, suffering from diabetes and taking insulin approached me. He wanted to know if hypnotherapy can help in controlling his diabetes as he did not want to take medicines for the whole life. He was perfectly healthy till two years back. Then his wife died of cancer, leaving him with the responsibility of looking after two daughters aged 18 and 21 alone and he suppressed his grief. The younger daughter was very much affected emotionally by the loss of mother and he was her sole support, as the elder daughter is married and living with her husband. When asked about his feelings he said that now he does not have any problem and he has adjusted well to the situation but wanted to stop insulin. He was taken into deep hypnosis and asked to observe the pancreas; he described the cells as unhealthy, the blood vessel clogged, and blood flow blocked and felt sad. I gave a suggestion to bring up the feelings and release them, and he started sobbing as he released the feelings. Then he became calm. Now he saw the blood flow to pancreas restored and cells recovering and he felt happy. After waking up he was surprised that he had so much emotional burden that he did not realize. After two more sessions his sugar level was controlled.

Internalization and accumulation of negative emotions can play a significant role in conditions like obesity, certain digestive disorders, insomnia, anaemia and cardiac diseases and kidney dysfunction.

Immunity related problems like immune deficiency syndrome can result from blockage of energy flow. Hypnotherapy employs a dual approach in treating such diseases, addressing the problem at the emotional and physical levels.

When emotions related to a particular reaction are repressed, they get accumulated in certain areas/organs of the body responsible for that reaction and later expressed as physical symptoms in that area. For example, a person wants to run away from a situation that he/she is unable to do. He/she feels frustrated and angry, but suppresses the feelings, which get repressed and stored in the modern memory. This may get expressed later as physical symptoms in the legs (the organs of escape) in the form of pain in the knees, ankles, etc.

> One of my friends Dr. Vandana, an Ayurveda doctor and hypnotherapist, told me about a patient she had treated. A 33 year old female came to her with severe anxiety, insomnia and recurring nightmares. She felt tired and lethargic. She has a 4 year old daughter. When some male cousin or male members of her husband's family caress the child she felt fear, anger and severe anxiety, with physical reactions like shivering, numbness in head, blurring of vision and nausea. She was taking medicines prescribed by her Psychiatrist for the last two years. During the pre-induction interview she had revealed that she was a victim of child abuse by her two cousins. After five sessions of hypnotherapy, in which stress reduction, releasing childhood trauma, anger and anxiety and building confidence were done, she became more confident and active and her anxiety and lethargy were totally gone. Her medicines were stopped. An unexpected outcome of the treatment was observed at the physical level. Some warts had developed in her hands during the last two years and she was planning to get them cauterized. These warts disappeared automatically when her emotional problems were resolved.

Her anger and anxiety regarding her daughter seem to have come from her own traumatic childhood experience. When the male members of the family caress her daughter, the subconscious memory of her childhood trauma triggered the reaction, which was expressed as anger, fear and anxiety and the accompanying physical symptoms. She had wanted to fight back, but could not do it, not even tell her parents and the feeling was suppressed. The warts were its physical expression in the hands, the organs of fight, which disappeared when the emotional problem was resolved. This is called **'body syndrome.'** Body syndromes can give a clue to the origin of some emotional symptoms.

How and why Hypnotherapy Works

The conventional methods of treatment of diseases focus on the physical symptoms. Symptoms are generally the signals to indicate that there is something not right there, that needs attention. For example, in many diseases pain is the signal coming from the subconscious mind to attract the attention of the conscious mind to the area of the problem for prompt remedial action. Remedy may not lie in relieving the pain only but needs to address the fundamental cause that created the pain. Therefore, treating the symptom alone may give relief from it, but will not cure the disease. One may use pain killers, which basically disconnect the transmitters of the pain signal to the brain. In many diseases, especially chronic conditions like diabetes, depression, hypertension, etc. the patient is advised to take medicines throughout life, because as the underlying emotional issue is not resolved the symptoms come back when the medicines are stopped. In order to get complete cure, there is a need to address the problem at the mental/emotional and physical levels. Support to this is coming from consciousness research, an emerging area of brain research. Studies by neuroscientists in some Universities in the USA and UK indicate that some mental health conditions like schizophrenia, obsessive compulsive disorder, depression, etc. might be caused by problems at the unconscious level or conflict between the conscious and unconscious pathways.

Hypnotherapy employs a holistic approach taking the body, mind and spirit together to ensure total health. It is based on the concept that all problems – physical, emotional and mental – originate in the mind. The healing also should come from the mind. The late Dr. Bernie Siegel, a famous British cancer surgeon and the author of the popular book *Love, Medicine and Miracles,* stated "there are no incurable diseases, only incurable people." Since hypnotherapy addresses the problem from the mind, the result once achieved remains for life.

It is important that the client remains relaxed to concentrate on the therapist's suggestion and respond properly. Studies have reported chemical changes in the body during deep relaxation; stress hormones like cortisol decreased and pleasure hormones like dopamine and serotonin levels were increased. People who understand hypnosis as an advanced form of relaxation easily accept it and benefit from it. People in deep somnambulistic stage benefit most from hypnotherapy, as they are highly receptive to verbal suggestions from the therapist and accept them as reality.

Chapter Seven
Visualization and Guided Imagery

Visualization

It is a method in which the person views an event or proceeding or action, as it is happening in front of him/her, i.e. creating a visual image of it in the mind.

I have often experienced the power of visualization on many occasions. There is also empirical evidence to show that visualization under deep concentration, done regularly and repeatedly, has similar effect as actual practice. I have used this technique whenever I have to give an important lecture in front of a large audience. The previous night, before going to sleep, I visualize the entire talk from start to finish, point by point, marking the time utilized on each point. This has always helped me to remember every point I want to present in the proper sequence and finishing it in the allotted time. Even physical changes can be brought about through focused visualization. A famous example of how visualization can heal physical problems is that of late Dr. Milton Erickson, a pioneer in modern hypnotherapy. He was afflicted by polio when he was 17 and the doctors who treated him declared that he is crippled for life without any hope of recovery and may not survive for more than 2-3 years. But he was not a person to give up so easily. Lying in bed with nothing else to do, he started visualizing each part of his body, imagining it regaining its health and function. By the age of 18 he completely recovered and joined the medical school and got his MD in Psychiatry. He contributed significantly to the development of hypnotherapy to the present level and getting it recognized by the American Medical Association. He died at the ripe old age of 79.

Positive visualization under hypnosis is very effective in bringing about positive changes in life. When you want to achieve something, with strong desire, firm resolve and conviction, positive visualization under self-hypnosis will help make it happen. This method is found to be effective in changing some attitudes and habits, self-improvement, improving stage performance, public speaking, interviews, sports etc. Everyone may not be able to visualize, but most people can imagine, which is found to be as effective as visualization when done under hypnosis.

For best results, each small detail from start to finish is visualized. For example, in athletics the person visualizes standing on the start line relaxed and confident, hearing the start signal, running with a feeling of winning, reaching the finish line much ahead of the others; and even standing on the victory stand, receiving the medal/trophy. This can be done under self-hypnosis, as it does not need very deep trance level. The visualization done 3–4 times a day, daily for a few weeks, is found to be effective. Under hetero hypnosis, the same results can be achieved in 3–4 sessions through guided imagery.

Guided Imagery

Here the therapist, after taking into deep hypnosis guides the client through every detail of the event/performance from start to finish, through verbal suggestions. I have found guided imagery a powerful method to get quick results in several areas.

> Angela, a 14 year old student was brought to me by her coach with a request to boost her confidence. She was participating in a National athletic meet. She was a good runner and was doing well in the practice sessions. But in the competitions, she became nervous and was not able to come up to the expected level. They had come on the previous evening. As the event was on the next morning, there was no time to lose; I agreed to do a session immediately. When I asked her about her problem, she said that while running she looks at the legs of the girl in front and feels that the other girl is faster, then she becomes nervous and loses confidence. She easily went

into deep hypnosis, and in that state first I gave a suggestion to build confidence. After that I did the guided imagery, in which she was asked to imagine standing herself at the start line; hearing the whistle to start and becoming relaxed and confident and start running with a winning feeling, focusing only on the track, everything else fading away, overtaking every other girl on the track; every time she overtakes someone her confidence increasing; reaching the finish line well ahead of the others, hearing the loud applause from the audience and her coach rushing towards her and giving her a big hug and she feeling wonderful and on top of the world. I repeated the visualization three times before waking her up. The next evening her coach informed me that she performed much better than what they expected and stood 4th in the order of finishing and broke her own previous record of time taken to complete the event.

Using triggers and anchors is very helpful in making the process effective. Trigger can be anything that the client does consciously, and anchor is the feeling that it generates. Relaxation, being a necessary pre-requisite for any performance, is a commonly used anchor. In the above example, I used the whistle (starting signal, gathered from talking to the coach) as the trigger and relaxation as anchor: "the moment you hear the whistle, you feel relaxed and confident and start running with a winning feeling" which were included in the suggestion. One may use other anchors like confidence, happiness, calmness, etc.

Guided imagery is found to be very useful in improving study habits and performance in examination, yielding remarkable results in 2–3 sessions. School students, appearing for Board examinations are found to benefit greatly from it.

Vishnu, a 16 year old boy, in 10th standard, was brought to me by his mother. He is intelligent and was a good student. But after his father died two years back, he was not paying attention to his studies; he had scored average marks in the model exam. Only one month left for the Board Examination, his mother was worried. Three sessions of hypnotherapy were done in one week. In the first session I gave a suggestion to improve study habits, followed by visualization of his studying daily, at a fixed time, for 3–4 hours with concentration, feeling good and enthusiastic about studies. In the second and third sessions, visualization also included a guided imagery of entering the examination hall and sitting in his allotted seat. Then I included a suggestion that the moment he takes the question paper in hand (trigger) he feels relaxed and confident (anchor) and all the information he has studied on the subject is recalled; and as he starts writing, the right answers to the questions come to his mind and he finishes answering all the questions correctly and in time, going home happy and with the firm resolve to continue studying with more effort and enthusiasm. He performed well in the Board examination and passed with high distinction marks, getting A-plus in 5 subjects, which his mother or teachers had not expected. He was so excited about the results that he immediately telephoned me to convey the good news.

For public speaking the suggestion could be "as you step on the podium/hold the mike (something the client usually does on such occasions), it will act as a trigger to make you relax and you become confident." Then take him/her through to the end of the speech, going home feeling happy and with a smile of satisfaction. Triggers and anchors can be used also in other situations like interviews, stage performance, acting, etc. Usually I repeat the guided imagery 3 times in one session. I have found three sessions are sufficient to get the desired effect in most cases. Each session can last from 45 to 60 minutes.

Hypnodrama

It is a guided imagery under hypnosis, usually employed for relationship issues: resolving interpersonal conflicts and misunderstandings. Interpersonal conflicts are, in most situations, because of preconceived distorted image or impression that a person entertains for another person. He/she responds to that distorted image of the other person rather than what he/she actually is. Some common examples are seen in issues between husband and wife, lovers, parent and child, employer and employee, sometimes even good friends. As the therapist, my effort is to bring out this distortion and help the client to smoothly act out the conflict in a safe environment, releasing the negative feelings and distorted associations. After taking the client into deep hypnosis, he/she is asked to visualize or imagine the other person sitting in a chair opposite him/her and express the disturbing feelings in words, speaking in the mind, releasing the feelings, then replace it with a positive feeling like love or happiness or peace. On waking up the person will feel more relaxed and calmer and with a changed attitude towards the other person.

Even one session of hypnodrama has been found to yield remarkable results in resolving some relationship issues.

> In one of my classes, there was a young lady, employed in a private company, who had problems with her boss. She was a sincere worker and the company had gained greatly through her projects. But she felt that her boss has been unfair to her when considering promotions and salary raises. She was very upset and angry and was thinking of quitting the job. She volunteered for the demo in the class. Under deep somnambulistic stage of hypnosis, I asked her to imagine her boss sitting in front of her and express her feelings verbally (in the mind). As she was following my suggestion, the bitterness and anger were evident on her face; she was tense in body, especially the right hand making a fist. Then she became relaxed and calm. On waking up she felt very relaxed and light. That one session was enough to resolve her issue with the boss. She informed me later that the next time she went to the office she explained everything calmly to her boss and was able to convince him; thereafter their relations became cordial and friendly.

Hypnodrama is similar to the Empty Chair technique used by psychologists. The advantage over the empty chair technique, which is done in the conscious state in the presence of the psychologist, is that in hypnodrama the client will not feel any inhibition in expressing the feelings, even if the hypnotherapist is present in the room, as everything is said and done in the mind. Moreover, he/she will be able to access the emotions buried deep in the subconscious mind (not possible in the conscious state) and release them. Compared to the Empty chair technique, hypnodrama gives faster and lasting results.

Role of Positive Thinking

> *'What we think that we are'*
>
> *– Lord Buddha*

Positive thinking is an essential ingredient of happiness. It is a skill that every one of us can develop consciously. Most people tend to look at the negative side of what happens in their life and surroundings. Continuous focusing on the negatives leads to a negative mindset and the person reaches a level that he/she cannot see anything positive. This can lead to frustration, helplessness, anxiety, depression, and even suicidal thoughts.

We must realize that only we are responsible for our experiences, because it is not the situation or the event itself, but how we view it and take it in with what types of feelings that counts. Some people remain confident and face the most adverse situations coolly and calmly, eventually coming out stronger, more energetic and confident. There are others who find even trivial things as insurmountable obstacles and lose all hope, going into dejection. A person with a negative mindset entertains pessimistic thoughts and feelings and is unable to think logically and in the right perspective. They run away from responsibilities, blaming others or the circumstances for their problem, leading to consequences that are self-destructive. Developing a positive mindset is what is needed to overcome such situations. Positive thinking can be developed by consciously trying to look at the positive side of unpleasant experiences and find out the lessons one can learn from it.

Regular practice of positive thinking helps in developing a positive mindset. A good example is stress. It is the manner in which one faces a situation that makes it stressful or not. People with a negative mindset view the situation with a defeatist attitude and gives up. A person with a positive mindset looks at the situation as a challenge and an opportunity to learn and faces it with confidence and determination. Hypnotherapy helps in changing the negative mindset, even releasing the negative feelings and replacing each feeling with a positive alternative and creating a more positive mindset.

Chapter Eight
Self Hypnosis

When I settled in Trivandrum some 15 years back, I found the city traffic in many places chaotic, traffic rules more evident in the number of times they are broken, vehicles rerouted into narrow side roads without any previous notice. I lost confidence in driving in the city. But I could not avoid it too as this is the city I had selected to spend the rest of my life. I used self-hypnosis and autosuggestion daily for about 3 weeks which removed my fear, and I became quite comfortable driving even on the narrow by-lanes.

Self-hypnosis is a method of taking oneself into a trance through autosuggestion. It is a state of deep concentration on one thing, word, or idea, excluding everything around. where one becomes less aware of the surroundings and more focused towards internal feelings. The conscious mind of the person himself/herself gives the suggestion to induce hypnosis. In hetero hypnosis the conscious mind hands over the control to the subconscious mind, whereas in self-hypnosis the conscious mind remains in control. But the information is allowed to bypass the analytical process and go directly into the subconscious mind. In that state the receptivity to self-suggestion increases, and therefore, easily accepted by the mind. But it cannot take a person very deep, only to a light trance, the hypnoidal stage.

Self-hypnosis is governed by the law of association and law of repetition. The state of relaxation is associated with an object or a sound or a word, which is repeated, taking the person gradually away from outside awareness into deep concentration inward. It is like the chanting of *"Aum"* or the rosary and the person going into a relaxed state of meditation.

All of us can use self-hypnosis and benefit from it. It can be used in many areas where one needs improvement, like building confidence, increasing concentration, overcoming shyness and timidity, improving study patterns and performing skills, taking initiative, changing some undesirable habits and attitudes that the person desires to achieve at a personal level, overcoming some fears like stage fear, fear of facing people, facing interviews, travelling, driving, etc. But it cannot be used for treatment of diseases.

> One of my clients, a young lady practitioner of Naturopathy, telephoned me one day; lately she had been feeling anxiety, low confidence and unable to take a decision in a very important matter concerning the whole family consisting of husband and two children. Since she was living about 250 km away and it was not possible for her to travel now, she wanted to know if I can suggest something to help her. I told her she can help herself and taught her a simple technique to do self-hypnosis. I asked her to do self-hypnosis and, in that state, to give a short suggestion in 2–3 sentences that she is confident of her ability to take the right decision and is happy and satisfied and her family is also happy with her decision, and repeat it 21 times every night before going to sleep for the next 3–4 weeks. About a month later she telephoned to tell me that after doing self-hypnosis and giving autosuggestion for two weeks she was able to take the decision and she and her husband are happy with it, because they know it is the best decision in the prevailing circumstances.

Autosuggestion followed by visualization under self-hypnosis is found to be more effective and yield faster results in areas where physical activity is involved. There are several examples of people who have benefited from self-hypnosis and autosuggestion and/or visualization in improving performance in interviews, seminars, stage presentation etc. For example, before going for a job interview, under self-hypnosis the person gives a suggestion to improve confidence, then visualizes the details of the interview from the preparation at home, sitting in the waiting hall, facing the experts, answering their questions with confidence, to finally leaving the room satisfied with the performance and feeling happy. The visualization repeated daily for a few days before the interview has been found to yield very positive results.

Self-hypnosis can be used successfully even in relieving some disturbing physical sensations like pain. I have been able to get relief from some muscular pains by visualization done under self-hypnosis.

> Once I was travelling by car; I was in the back seat with two other persons. It was a 6–7 hours journey. After about a couple of hours I developed acute pain in my lower back. I did not want to disturb the others. So, I closed my eyes and went into a light trance. Then I visualized the pain as a small stone pressing into my back muscle, which I pulled out and threw away into the distance, making it disappear. As the stone gained distance, I felt the pain becoming less and completely gone with the disappearance of the stone.

The stone was a symbol of the feeling of pain, created by the subconscious mind; so, removing the symbol was accepted as releasing the feeling and it became the reality. Similar experience has been narrated by one of my students.

Visualization under self-hypnosis is found to benefit patients recovering from physical handicaps, but it is a slow process and will need several sessions through an extended period of days or even months. The most famous example is that of Dr. Milton Erickson (given in the previous chapter), who recovered from polio related physical disability through daily visualization. In some clients who need multiple sessions, after a few sessions with me I teach self-hypnosis and ask them to do self-hypnosis at home and visualise under that state the desired changes happening, daily during the period between sessions. I have found visualizing under hypnosis beneficial in accelerating the recovery process, especially in patients paralysed on one side due to stroke or brain injury.

> A patient undergoing physiotherapy in the palliative care centre in Thrissur was referred to me. He was paralysed on the right side and his right hand and leg were immobile. I took him into deep hypnosis and asked him to visualize his small toe on the right leg lifting up, first gradually and then to the possible maximum height; after a few sessions when improvement was seen in that toe, I asked him to do the same with the other toes, one by one, repeating several times with each toe. After 3 sessions I taught him how to go into a light trance and asked him to do the process at home under the trance state, several times daily till the next session which was after one month. When I saw him next, he was able to move the small toe more freely and the toe next to it was also more flexible. This was possible because he was following my instruction sincerely and doing the exercise regularly.

The change is slow, and it can take several weeks, even months, before noticeable improvement occurs. It needs patience and regular practice to get the desired effect. In the above case, recovery of the whole leg could be achieved, but it will take one year or more with continuous practice by the client several times daily at home with a monthly session with me (the therapist). But in most cases, the clients lose patience and give up after a few days, because they are expecting miraculous changes in a few sessions, which is not possible in such cases. Unlike in emotional problems, where a couple of sessions can produce noticeable effect, physical changes can take months before the effect starts to show. So, with a strong resolve to change and regular practice, it is possible to achieve improvement in many areas at the personal level through self-hypnosis.

For the benefit of the readers who may like to use self-hypnosis for personal improvement, I have given a couple of methods below. More methods can be found on the net. But I think a few words of caution are in place here.

1. It is not advised to do self-hypnosis when a person is depressed or in a very negative mood or feeling very low or sad, or while driving.

2. It is better to keep the suggestion short and simple, so that it will be easy to remember and repeat under hypnosis.

3. Only one issue may be taken at a time. Mixing up issues or clubbing together of many issues can be ineffective. If more than one issue is being handled, it will be best to give separate suggestion for each issue, waking yourself up after giving one suggestion; hypnotise again and give the second suggestion and then wake yourself up, repeating this process for each issue.

4. Best effects are obtained when the suggestion is repeated several times, 21 times is recommended, in one session daily for several days.

5. It is very important to wake oneself up at the end of the session.

Method 1

Sit straight in a semi-comfortable chair with head supported or on a recliner. It can also be done in lying position, but then the head should be raised one foot.

Select any point on the wall in front or, if lying position, on the ceiling, fix your eyes on that point and keep staring at it.

Focus on your breathing, feeling the breath coming in and going out. Breathe in through the nose and breathe out through the mouth; imagine releasing negative energy and taking in positive energy. After 5–7 breaths, breathe normally through the nose, concentrating on the breath. Feel the eye lids growing heavy and starting to close.

Gently close your eyes and feel the relaxation in the eyelids. Realise it, become one with it.

Visualize or imagine or feel the relaxation spreading from the eyelids, to the cheeks and chin, feel the jaw muscles relaxing; let the relaxation spread up the forehead, the scalp, down the neck and throat, relaxing every muscle.

Imagine or feel the relaxation spreading to the shoulders, down the hands to the tips of the fingers; feel the hands growing limp and heavy, deeply relaxing.

Let the relaxation slowly spread down to the upper back, all the way down to the tip of the spine, relaxing all the muscles in the back, just like a mental massage. Enjoy the feeling, relaxing deeper and deeper.

Allow the relaxation to spread to the chest area and abdomen, down through the hips, thighs, all the way down to the tips of the toes.

Once again focus on the relaxation, feel it completely saturating the whole body, from the top of the head to the tips of the toes; feel calm and peaceful as you continue to relax more and more with every breath.

Now say in your mind: 'I am going to count myself down from 5 to 0, with every count I will feel more relaxed and calm, going deeper and deeper and at 0, when I say "deep sleep" I will enter a deep hypnotic state and my body will be fully relaxed; 5, 4, 3, 2, 1, 0, deep sleep.'

Now you can give the suggestion that you have prepared for the change you desire. Repeat the suggestion 21 times.

Continue breathing normally, focusing on your breath for about a couple of minutes and then wake yourself up by saying 'I am going to count myself up from 1 to 5, I will be fully awake at 5, feeling relaxed and good, 1, 2, 3, 4 and 5, wide awake.' Open your eyes and feel comfortable.

Method 2

Sit comfortably in a chair or recliner. Take a few deep breaths, focusing on your breath, breathe out all tension and breathe in relaxation.

Gently close your eyes and breathe normally, focusing on your breath. Continue for some time, feeling more and more relaxed with every breath and your attention completely focused on your breath.

Visualize or imagine yourself in a beautiful garden, walking alone on a path in the garden. You are surrounded by the garden; feel yourself enjoying the walk, watching the flowers, trees, noticing the beautiful colours of the flowers, feeling their fragrance in the air, feeling the cool, refreshing, calming breeze caressing your face, becoming more and more relaxed.

At the end of the path, see or imagine a staircase and now you are standing on top of the staircase. The staircase has 15 steps leading down. You are feeling very relaxed as you stand on top of the staircase.

Say to yourself 'I am going to count from 15 down to 0 and I will go down the staircase taking one step down with each count, feeling 10 times more relaxed with each step I take down, and by the count of 0, as I reach the bottom of the staircase, I will be in a very deep state of relaxation.'

Count slowly: 15…14…13…12…11…10…9…8…7…6…5…4…3…2…1…0 and say 'deep sleep.'

Now give the suggestion you have prepared. Repeat the suggestion 21 times.

Wait for about a couple of minutes, breathing normally; then wake yourself up by saying to yourself 'I am going to count myself up from 1 to 5; I will be fully awake at 5, feeling relaxed and good; 1, 2, 3, 4, 5, wide awake.' Open your eyes, feel comfortable.

Note: It is advisable to do self-hypnosis in an assigned place and time. You can choose any time according to your convenience, but the last half hour before going to sleep, the so-called 'magic 30 minutes,' is a good time to do self-hypnosis, as the suggestion will be processed first and stored in its full strength.

Chapter Nine
Regression Therapy

*Arjuna, you and I have passed through many births.
I know them all, but you do not know.*

– *Bhagavad Gita, Chapter 4, Verse 5.*

'I am in a battlefield. There are bodies all around, bodies of dead soldiers.' Suddenly her expression changed, showing distress, intense pain. She said repeatedly 'I am bleeding... I am dying,' then became quiet and her face became calm.

This was a young girl of 16, under deep hypnosis, undergoing hypnotherapy to remove her fear of blood. She had regressed back to a life when she was a soldier in the Second World War.

Regression therapy is based on the concept that many of our present problems have their origin in some traumatic experiences earlier either in this life or in a past life. In such cases we take the person to the origin of the problem, wherever it is, experience the event and the associated feelings and remove them from the root. This is done in regression therapy. Resolving the issue in the past will have the same effect as removing the problem in the present. Regression therapy is not discussed in detail here, only a brief introduction is given, as it is not in the scope of this book.

There are two types of regression:

- past life regression where a person goes to a previous lifetime.
- age regression where the client goes to an earlier age in the present life.

Past Life Regression

The person under deep hypnosis is guided through suggestions to an event in a past life which has the cause of origin of the problem and the healing is done there. Healing at the origin will resolve the problem in the present. This is called Past Life Regression Therapy (PLRT).

PLRT is based on the concept of reincarnation and the belief that we take birth again and again to resolve unresolved karmic issues and learning lessons from those experiences, which is needed for the evolution of the soul to higher energy levels. Concept of Karma and rebirth are an integral part of Hindu philosophy.

> The 16 year old girl mentioned in the beginning of the chapter, Bela was brought to me by her mother. She had some study problem, which was corrected through a couple of hypnotherapy sessions, with suggestions to improve the study habits. Then her mother said Bela has an unreasonable fear of blood. She was so scared of seeing blood, that she did not allow even routine blood tests. The sight of blood in movies on a TV screen made her panicky, with giddiness and even fainting. I took her into deep hypnosis and guided through suggestion to the origin of her fear of blood. She saw herself as a soldier in Hitler's army, in a battlefield in the second World War, with dead bodies strewn around her. She was shot in the chest and died there. The last words she uttered were 'I am bleeding, I am dying.' As she was describing the scene her expression changed to one of distress and pain and tears rolled down her cheeks. Her fear of blood was carried forward from that experience where she associated bleeding with death. After the session she lost her fear and even volunteered to test her mother's blood for diabetes.

Past Life Regression is not a simple memory recall, which is the function of the conscious mind. The person relives the event, actually feeling all the traumas, injury, pain, emotions like grief, fear, anger, etc. that he/she experienced at that time. The therapist can observe the change in facial expressions, muscles stiffening, tears flowing down from the eyes, sobbing and other reactions as the person describes the experience.

Several chronic conditions like many phobias, asthma, psoriasis, some unexplainable pains, and panic attacks have been traced back to some past life events, where PLRT gave lasting relief. A few cases from my experience are cited below as empirical evidence.

> A police constable in his early 30s experienced an intense fear while facing crowds; his muscles becoming tight and body sweating profusely, and he was unable to think or react properly. There was no reason for his extreme reaction known to him. He was a well-built man, physically fit and serving in the police force for some years, the most unlikely person to have such a problem. Under deep hypnosis he was guided to the origin of his fear and he regressed to a life about 100 years back. He was a senior minister in the king's court, responsible for bringing reformations and development of the rural sector. He had some innovative ideas that he wanted to implement, but some groups of people were against it. He had called a meeting of the cabinet and invited the leaders of those groups as he wanted to explain the plan and convince the people about its benefits. When he started the discussion some of the group leaders got up, there were arguments, and this minister was dragged down and beaten to death. In the present life as a policeman he had to face crowds and control the mob. The sight of crowds triggered the subconscious memory of that event of about 100 years back, unknown to his conscious mind, causing his reactions. Reliving the experience and releasing the fear from there resolved his present problem.

In some cases, repetition of similar experiences through different rebirths has been observed. Rebirths could be in different countries, different religious faiths, and can be as man or woman.

> One of my clients, a lady in her early 60s, a retired school teacher, was suffering from severe asthma for many years. She was taking medicines, using inhaler and nebulizer, but the frequent attacks were making even routine activities difficult. She had read a book by Dr. Brian Weiss, the famous hypnotherapist and popular author of many books on past life therapy and approached me as she wanted to try it. I told her it can take several sessions and she may not go to a past life in the first session and she agreed. After explaining hypnotherapy and past life therapy, I took her into deep hypnosis and gave suggestion to reduce tension. On waking up she felt good and relaxed and said it was a good experience. We fixed further sessions during the following weeks in which PLRT was done. She went through five different lifetimes, going back through centuries in different places and different circumstances, as woman or man; in each one of them death was due to suffocation. The first lifetime she went was about 200 years back in a European country. She is a

beautiful princess and her wedding preparations are in progress. The whole kingdom is in a festive mood. But on the day of her wedding her younger sister, who is in love with the groom, offers her a sweet dish lazed with a strong poison and she dies. The last sensations before she dies are those of choking, suffocation and breathlessness. In an earlier life she saw herself as a young man, waiting for his friend near a forest. A fire breaks out, destroying the whole forest and he dies of suffocation due to the smoke from the fire. In another life again she is a young woman, living with her mother. Their house collapses in a storm and the wall falls on her, crushing her chest and suffocating her to death; she used to get pain in the chest which disappeared after this session. In an earlier life she is a woman with a boat, catching fish; the boat capsizes, and she is drowned. Then she went to the first time, the origin of her present breathing problem, a life as a woman. It is a prehistoric scenario, a community of people sitting around a big fire in a clearing in the forest, cooking some animals the men have hunted, by hanging them on a pole above the fire. They have covered the lower part of the body with grass. There are no houses, people live in caves. She had gone to the forest to fetch firewood. As she returns through the forest she is bitten by a poisonous snake. The poison spreads in her body, she is unable to breathe and dies of suffocation. With each session she got some relief, and gradually reduced the medicines and use of inhaler. After the last session where she lived in the forest and died of snake bite, her condition improved so much, she could completely stop the use of nebulizer and inhaler. Now it is almost 5 years after her last session. She is quite happy, her quality of life increased beyond her expectations.

In more than 90% of asthma cases, death due to suffocation in previous lives is found to be the root cause. In the above case she had gone to each life in a sequential order. But I have seen some clients going directly to the original event, even centuries back.

One of my clients was an Ayurveda doctor, 27 years old lady. As long as she could remember she had been in and out of hospitals, subjected to different treatments for emotional and physical problems like anxiety, depression, claustrophobia, breathing difficulty, choking feeling, thyroid disorder, and bleeding from skin, nose, etc., immune deficiency and several other clinical symptoms. She felt pain in all joints, and it was difficult to sit for long, which was affecting her practice as an Ayurveda doctor. The doctors treating her had reached the conclusion that nothing more can be done, and she must live with the problems. That is when she approached me. In the first session, she was confused and could not tell me what issue she wants to address first. She went into deep hypnosis very fast. I gave suggestions to reduce stress and release negative feelings. When she came for the second session, she was clearer about her priorities and said she would like to start with her thyroid problem. I took her into a deep somnambulistic stage, and she regressed back to a life more than 1000 years ago, to an event which was the original cause of her problem. In that life she saw herself as a 17 year old girl in a long silk skirt and blouse, attending a function with her mother. She is standing near a fireplace, in which the priests are trying to destroy some very poisonous material by burning it. Some of the poison falls on her foot and gradually spreads up, paralyzing each part, and blood is oozing out from the skin and different parts of the body. As the poison spreads to the chest, breathing becomes difficult and she feels suffocated. She is transferred to a separate hut and Vaidyas (doctors) are trying to treat her with herbs, without success. Then, as the final act of destroying the poison, they burn the hut with her inside. She could see her dead body with blisters due to burning. After removing the trauma and healing the body, I brought her back to the present and woke her up. She felt very relaxed and her body pain had completely gone. She recovered from her problems without further sessions and stopped taking medicines, as she wanted to see how much hypnotherapy has done for her. After 3 months she telephoned me to tell that 90% of her problems are gone, her thyroid tests showed normal values, bleeding has stopped, joint pain, breathing difficulty and claustrophobia have completely disappeared and she is comfortable sitting in the clinic for hours together. Now it is more than 2 years after that session, and she is quite happy that she opted for hypnotherapy.

Sometimes the same people may come together in different lifetimes, but relationships can be different. Those who have karmic connections are born as contemporaries and brought together at some or other time of life, as a part of the plan in the life script.

An interesting case I treated is that of a 30 year old lady, an only child, married a year back to the man of her choice. They are a happy couple, living with her parents. One day her husband went to his parents' house, at a distance of 2 hours drive, telling her that he will be back by the evening. He could not return the same day, so he telephoned and informed her that he will come back the next day. She became very upset and started crying, saying that she is abandoned, and nobody is there for her. She kept wailing loud the whole night and the parents could not console her. She became quiet only when her husband returned the next morning.

Her parents brought her to me because they were worried about how she may behave again when her husband goes out for some work. As I was taking her deep into hypnosis, she started showing distress. When asked what is troubling her, she said her husband has gone to another town and has not come back. She had regressed back to a previous lifetime. She is a young woman living with her husband and his parents. They live in a village in Kerala. Her husband had gone to Madras in search of a job some days back. He has not returned and there is no news about him. She is worried that something must have happened to him. She and his parents keep waiting for months, the hope of his returning diminishing. She feels lonely, sad, always thinking of him, becomes mentally deranged and commits suicide. In the present incidence when her husband informed that he will not come back as promised, the memory of that life was triggered, bringing up the feelings that she experienced in that life. She also identified her husband in that lifetime as the same person as her present husband. After waking up she was amused about how she had overreacted in the present situation.

Age Regression

Childhood experiences can play a significant role in moulding our behaviour as an adult. Since children function at the subconscious level, everything they experience, good and bad, are stored with 100% intensity in the modern memory. Painful memories can lead to behavioural disorders later in life; many fears like fear of dogs, fear of spider, etc. are found to have origin in the childhood. Treatment is done under very deep hypnosis by regressing back to the original event at a younger age in the present life and releasing the feeling from there.

The following example can illustrate this. A 47 year old company executive approached me with a respiratory problem; he often gets choking feeling, as if something is blocking the air flow. Clinical tests did not show any abnormality or pathological changes. He told me that he felt that some poisonous gas is in his lungs, causing the problem, but the tests are not able to detect it. I asked him if he could recall any such experiences earlier. He said that when he was in the school, he used to go to the chemical factory owned by his elder brother and once he accidentally inhaled some poisonous gas. Immediately he was taken to the hospital and recovered completely after treatment. He had no health problems after that and at 47 he is maintaining good physical health, but he gets recurring feeling of choking. He has undergone all tests several times, which gave normal results.

Under deep hypnosis, he was asked to go to the origin of his choking feeling. He regressed back to an event in his early teens; he is in his brother's factory and accidentally one of the storage cans is opened and he inhales the gas, starts respiratory distress and choking feeling. In that stage of hypnosis anything can be imagined which is accepted as reality by the mind. I asked him to examine his respiratory passage and see what is causing the problem. He saw a green slimy object sticking to the windpipe blocking the air flow. I asked him to imagine him removing the object and clearing the area and the air flow became smooth. After waking up he felt good. After that session he never got the choking feeling again.

In this case, even though the treatment immediately after he inhaled the gas in the childhood had removed the toxic gas from the system, his mind had stored it as a threat (the green slimy object was the symbol of that toxin) and was sending a warning signal to the conscious mind, and that was being expressed as the choking sensation. Under regression, the mind cleared the system of that object from its origin, which the subconscious mind accepted as the reality, resolving his problem.

There are cases where a person regressed back to the foetal stage.

In a class while doing a demonstration of anger release, the subject, a lady in her early 50s, regressed to the time when she was in the womb of her mother, an 8 month old foetus. She described the scenario where her father is angrily shouting and beating her mother and she feels angry and sad, at the same time, helpless. She started sobbing while describing it. I helped her, through suggestion, to release the anger and replace it with love and forgiveness, and the bitterness towards her father and anger left her.

On waking up, she was surprised at her reaction under hypnosis, as she was not aware of her internalized feelings. In most cases, after waking up, the person can remember what they experienced and said when under hypnosis.

In age regression, the person is going back to an event that happened at an early age in the present life, into the modern memory. So, the chances of installing false memory cannot be ruled out. Therefore, the therapist must be careful not to give any negative suggestions nor ask leading questions, which can create false memory. As you are addressing the subconscious mind, which accepts everything without analysing or filtering, it will be stored in the modern memory and can lead to new problems. Therefore, age regression is used as a last resort, when the other methods like desensitization, guided imagery, hypnodrama, etc. fail to yield satisfactory result.

PLRT is safer than age regression and more within the defence safeguards; and chances of creating false memories are very rare as we are going to the primitive memory, to something which happened in another life, another time and another body.

Part II
Applications of Hypnotherapy

Chapter Ten

Introduction

Now that you have a basic idea about hypnosis and hypnotherapy, we can move on to their applications in human health.

Hypnotherapy is used as a complementary and alternative therapy in several hospitals in USA and UK. But it is not yet accepted as a clinical possibility in India, where it still falls into the category of miracles or magic or even hallucination. It is a fact that most problems handled under psychotherapy and psychiatry are amenable to hypnotherapy; the results are faster and more lasting. Tremendous success and lasting relief have been obtained in different health issues. Several cases from the personal experience of the author, cited in this book, clearly show the wide areas of its application in human health care. These include non-clinical, mainly emotional and behavioural issues; clinical, diagnosed as mental and physical diseases; other health conditions which are natural, like child birth, but where clinical intervention may be required; and behavioural and other problems in children. In the emotional issues hypnotherapy gives fast results; in some chronic mental conditions and physical diseases changes take longer, 3-6 months or more may be needed to get satisfactory results.

Most of the clients who seek my help are those who have tried other methods of treatment or counselling; they come with a fixation of their problem, inferred from the clinical diagnosis, collected from internet, or heard from other people, who may have only a superficial knowledge about such things. For example, the general belief that if you have chronic diseases like diabetes, hypertension, asthma, depression, etc., the treatment is lifelong. In the case of cancers, many people do not know that most cancers are curable if diagnosed and treated in the early stages; the word 'cancer' is taken as the death knell and treatment is feared due to the anticipated side effects.

As mentioned earlier in this book, hypnotherapy does not go by the medical diagnosis, which is based on physical and physiological parameters. Our treatment is based on the client's/patient's perception of the problem/disease, his/her feelings and mental image of the problem, as impressed in the subconscious mind. The purpose of treatment is to change that perception from an unhealthy to a healthy state, from negative to positive, making the person happy and satisfied. Once the mind accepts the change, it works to make it the reality by creating the circumstances and facilities needed to change the physiological, physical and mental aspects accordingly. Each cell has its own consciousness, memory and intelligence, which work together to bring about the changes needed to create the healthy state. But the healing depends on the karmic debt that is to be resolved. The change can occur only if the mind views the time as right. Every disease has a purpose, to remind you of something or to learn from that experience. For serious health issues, before attempting treatment, I try to find out from the person under hypnosis if it is time to resolve the issue and if it is the right time to treat. If the answer is in the negative, then hypnotherapy may not help in healing, but can have a palliative effect.

> A 63 year old house wife was brought to me by her daughter. She had joint pains and body pain. She was taking medicines for some time without much benefit. They were in Trivandrum, where I am based, to consult another doctor for a second opinion and approached me to see if I can help in relieving the pain. I fixed the session at 10 the next morning, as her appointment with the new doctor was in the afternoon. Under deep hypnosis I asked her if it is time for her to resolve her problem and what she has to do for it. She said that it can be cured, but the medicines that she is taking now have to be changed. When she met the doctor in the afternoon he said that the earlier diagnosis was wrong and changed the medicines, which benefited her.

This lady had only a basic school education and had spent her whole life in a remote village and would not have known anything about the medical aspects. But the mind knows what is good for us and the right time to take the right action.

In another case, where I treated a 48 year old lady suffering from chronic depression, after several sessions in which different emotional problems were addressed, even though she became active and cheerful, some unknown fear was still nagging her. The origin of this fear was found to be in a past life, which was resolved through regression therapy. I asked her subconscious if it is time now to be free from those bindings, it said that she has paid her debt through the long suffering and she need not suffer any more. After that session only two more sessions were needed to achieve catharsis. This was about 9 years back. Since then she is leading a happy and peaceful life.

Hypnotherapy has found its application in almost all areas of human health, and is applicable in all age groups, without any contra-indications or side effects. The different areas of its application are listed in Table 1. Some specific areas include Cancer therapy, Surgery, Obstetrics, Dentistry, Physiotherapy, Geriatrics, and Palliative care.

Table 1: Areas of Application of Hypnotherapy

- Anxiety
- Asthma
- Addictions – alcohol, drugs
- Anger
- Anorexia
- Anxiety
- Bed wetting
- Bereavement
- Burns
- Career improvement
- Child abuse
- Compulsive eating
- Concentration enhancement
- Confidence building
- Delivery
- Depression
- Diabetes
- Divorce
- Dyslexia
- Eating disorders
- Examinations
- Fears – all types
- Guilt perception
- Headaches
- Hypertension
- Hypochondria
- Immune disorders
- Immunity boosting
- Impotence
- Inferiority complex
- Insecurity feeling
- Insomnia
- Irritable bowel syndrome
- Jealousy
- Memory improvement
- Migraines
- Mood changes
- Obesity
- Obsessive compulsive disorder
- Overeating
- Pains – all types
- Panic
- Performance anxiety
- Personality development
- Phobias – all types
- Premature ejaculation
- Procrastination
- Public speaking
- Relationship issues
- Relaxation
- Sadness
- Self confidence
- Self esteem
- Sexual problems
- Nail biting
- Nausea
- Skin problems
- Sleep disorders
- Smoking
- Social phobia
- Sports performance
- Stage fright
- Stammering
- Stress control
- Study habits
- Substance abuse
- Tardiness
- Thumb sucking
- Timidity
- Traumas
- Twitches
- Ulcers
- Weight loss
- Writer's block

Some of the applications are discussed in more detail, with examples from case studies, in the following chapters. Some cases were already discussed in the earlier chapters.

Chapter Eleven

Nonclinical Applications

Many problems for which the clients approach me are not clinically categorized as diseases. These are viewed as behavioral or emotional issues, which the person is not able to manage and for which they seek professional help. Some of them are described in more detail below.

Stress Management

It is often said that stress is one of the most destructive elements in people's daily lives, but that is only half truth. The way we react to stress appears to be more important than stress itself.

– Bernie Siegel

Ajitha, a 43 year old, single, working lady approached me for help in controlling stress. She is sincere and hard working. She has a lot of stress and anxiety and is low in confidence. She feels that others are taking advantage of her and she does not get credit for what she does; no one listens to her, while she accepts the burden and gives space to others. She wants to fight back but is not able to. She was even thinking of quitting her job. That is when she sought my help.

She had a traumatic childhood. Her mother was working elsewhere and when she was seven, she was left to live with her maternal grandparents and uncle and his wife, who did not give her love. Her teenage years also were not happy, she was compared with her cousins who were more beautiful than her. Three sessions of hypnotherapy were done, in which suggestions were given for stress reduction, confidence building and goal achievement. She became relaxed, more confident and more open about her feelings.

Stress poses a serious threat to normal life and functioning, especially in the modern scenario, where every individual of every age is under one or other type of stressful condition. Constant stress results in emotional and behavioral issues like irritation, anger, intolerance, frustration, and helplessness, that, in the long run, can lead to mental problems and physical disorders. Most of the time the clients do not recognize stress as the cause of their irritation, frustration, anger, insomnia, etc. for which they seek professional help. Therefore, it is important to maintain a stress-free condition for a healthy life. Stress control is the most sought after application of hypnotherapy in the corporate world.

> Sukumar, a 29 year old Software engineer, is over-stressed. He is unmarried and is staying with his parents; he wants to live independently but does not have a secure job. Parents are always arguing, and keep advising him regarding his food and expenses, and mother is nagging, which creates more stress. When under stress he loses self-control and over-eats, which makes him more stressed and he loses confidence. He felt that he is slipping into depression. He came to me seeking help in overcoming stress and anxiety and to have control over his eating. Four sessions of hypnotherapy were done, with 2 days gap between sessions, in which suggestions for stress reduction, removing anxiety and depression and building self-confidence were given; guided imagery for changing food habit to a healthier and controlled diet was also done in 2 sessions. That took care of his stress and anxiety and he became more relaxed and able to regulate his food intake.

All of us are surrounded by stressful situations and nobody can avoid them, as they are a part of modern life. It is not stress itself, but the manner in which one handles the situation that decides if it is stressful or not. For some people, stress acts as a positive stimulus, motivating them to look for methods to overcome it and emerge out more confident and successful. But for most people stress has a negative influence. Childhood conditioning can have a significant role in deciding how a person is equipped to cope with stressful situations, as is evident in the example of Ajitha cited above.

> I treated a 23 year old student, staying away from home in the hostel, who complained of tension, lack of confidence, and lack of concentration in studies. She also was afraid of facing audience, had difficulty in presenting seminars, etc. She had attempted suicide twice when she was in 5th or 6th standard. Two sessions of hypnotherapy were done with a gap of one week between sessions, in which negative feelings were released, desensitization to feelings experienced in the situation of tension (stress) was done, followed by suggestion to build confidence. She became tension-free and confident and started interacting with friends more freely.

Stress weakens the immune system and stops the experience of joy. It is a reaction of the autonomic nervous system and not in the control of the brain. All of us have all the resources and capability to face stressful situations calmly and overcome them efficiently. But many of us are not trained for that or are unable to use them, may not even be aware of our inherent resources. Hypnotherapy helps to discover our inner potentials and strengths and use them effectively for our benefit. This is done by the therapist through suggestions given under hypnosis, desensitizing to the stress inducing situations and building self-confidence, leading to self-awakening and empowerment, so that the person is able to recognize and release it, and utilize his/her inherent potentials to bring about the desired changes in attitude.

In some cases, childhood trauma is found to be at the base of the stress.

> Madhavi, an Engineering graduate, not employed, consulted me for stress, anxiety, anger and tension. Her husband is in Gulf and she is staying in Kerala with her in-laws. She is not able to accept her mother-in-law. In the first two sessions, stress reduction and release of anger towards mother-in-law were done and tension reduced. In the third session, desensitization to anger in general was done. Even though she became more relaxed and was able to control her anger and better accept her mother-in-law, there was some tension and fear which she could not explain. In the next session, under deep somnambulistic stage, I asked her to go to the origin of her problem. She regressed back to age 3; she is in the bedroom with her parents and grandparents. Her father is angry and shouting and she becomes tense and feels scared, which were released. After that session, her tension and fear disappeared, which points to the origin of the

present problem in the childhood, which explains why treating the present state alone was not able to give complete relief.

Personality Development

Many of the clients who approach me for personal improvement are found to be in a confused state of mind and are not able to tell exactly what they want. Some of the specific areas where they need improvement are self-confidence, motivation, specific goal setting and commitment; these are brought out during the pre-induction interview.

> Manish, a 32 year old Educational Advisor, presented with lack of clarity of mind, lack of concentration and poor memory, and inability to complete the assigned tasks. He has been taking psychiatric medicines for the last 4 years. When he does not take medicine, he feels angry, then he gets headache and rumbling in the stomach. He was lethargic, not able to enjoy TV or music, which he used to do earlier. His sleep was disturbed, and he felt tired on waking up in the morning.
>
> Four sessions of hypnotherapy were done; during the first two sessions suggestion to remove depression, followed by suggestion to build confidence was given. He became more relaxed and cheerful, started watching TV and became active in face book group in which he had lost interest, and was sleeping better, but still was unable to concentrate. In the next session, suggestions to increase concentration and confidence were given in the 4th session, done after one week, his work potential was increased by a method called Transcript of Life therapy, raising his unconscious script from a level of 4 to 8 (This is a method developed by John Kappas, where under deep hypnosis a person's potential in the area of interest is increased through suggestions; once the subconscious mind accepts it, it helps to change all aspects of the person's life to make it a reality). He came after 3 weeks, very happy. He said that now he has clarity of mind, confidence has increased, he is able to do things with responsibility, able to concentrate, confident of writing on any topic he selects; performance level and memory also increased. He did not want another session.

Confidence building is an important part of personality development. Repeated experiences of frustrating incidences in life can create a defeatist attitude. Moreover, to a great extent, how one is treated in childhood and in school determines the way he/she is groomed and prepared to face adverse circumstances. A child hearing negative comments repeatedly from the parents, caretakers or teachers gets demoralised and loses self-confidence and develops a negative image of himself/herself and grows up thinking that he/she is good for nothing. The person starts doubting himself/herself, losing self-confidence and self-esteem, leading to frustration, anger, feeling worthless and hopeless and gets demoralised. They feel that whatever they do is going to fail and hence stop trying, shrink away from responsibilities and lose purpose in life. A strong personality enables the person to face adverse situations with confidence and equanimity. Proper suggestions given under hypnosis help build confidence and increase self-esteem and bring awareness of the hidden talents, motivating the person to use his/her potentials fully, develop optimism and positive attitude towards life and prepare him/her to face any situation as a challenge and an opportunity to learn and progress.

> A 40 year old man, a clerk in a government office, approached me for improving confidence and speed in work. During the pre-induction interview, it turned out that he has a lot of anxiety and fear and was under tension related to job and his sleep was disturbed; he felt drowsy while in the office. Three sessions of hypnotherapy were done, in which tension and anxiety were released and suggestion to build confidence was given. After 2 sessions, he became relaxed, felt more confident and was able to concentrate on work and was sleeping better. One more session was done after 2 weeks and suggestions to increase concentration and confidence were given and his problem was resolved.

Thus, personality development is not improving just one thing like confidence or self-esteem but needs to address different aspects at the mental and emotional levels and physical activity, which can take a few sessions, but it is found to be rewarding.

Anger

> Chandana, a 38 year old Nursing Assistant, living with her husband and 2 year old daughter, approached me seeking help to control anger. She gets angry when someone talks to her when she is in a stressed state, or others do not listen to her. Then she talks loudly,

shouts, and sometimes even explodes. She had anger problem since she was 8 years or so, but lately it was getting out of control. Three sessions of hypnotherapy were able to produce satisfactory results.

Bharath, 28 years old man, who holds a postgraduate degree in Business Management, quit his job in the Gulf as he could not adjust there; now he is working as a Sales agent. He gets angry when his parents object to something he says, gets agitated and shouts. He also was afraid of facing people. He had consulted a psychiatrist and taken medicines 3 years back, but it gave relief for a short time. Four sessions of hypnotherapy were done, and his anger and fear were controlled.

Anger is a common issue for which people from all fields and of all ages approach me for help. Uncontrolled anger is very detrimental to a healthy life. When angry, a person loses all logic and behaves impulsively, and says or does things that he/she may not do under normal state of mind. This creates problems at home, workplace and in society, affecting family life, job security and social standing. Family atmosphere, where other members are non-empathetic, can aggravate the problem.

Bindu, a 19 year old final year school student was brought to me by her parents. She was not taking interest in studies and gets angry at parents when they ask her to study or scold her for not studying. She was class leader when she was in 10th std. When the other students refused to obey her, she became angry; when the teacher scolded her she reacted violently. Then she was taken to a psychiatrist and was admitted for 2 weeks in the psychiatrist ward and treated with medicines. After that she was under Ayurveda treatment for some time. She was taking homeopathy medicines when she came to me. Family atmosphere was also not helping; her parents did not understand her and always criticized her. Two sessions of hypnotherapy were done, in which anger was released and replaced with feeling of happiness. Her anger was controlled, and her healing was faster with a change in atmosphere; she shifted to her elder sister's house, where she was more comfortable and happy. She had developed an attachment with a boy and wanted to get married immediately, but her parents were against it and wanted her to study and get a good job before thinking of marriage, which was also a reason for her behavioral problem. After the anger was controlled, she considered the issue again and wanted to be emotionally free from that attachment, which was done in the 3rd session and she became more cheerful and serious about her studies.

Some angers have their origin in the childhood or even in the prenatal life (as in the case of the class demo, described in chapter 9).

> A 35 year old housewife, living with husband, a businessman and teenage son, sought my help in controlling anger. She was married at the age of 17. Her anger became a problem after marriage. When angry she shouts at her husband and son, sometimes breaks things; in extreme situations she feels like committing suicide. There was some fear also associated with the anger episodes. She had a difficult childhood, lived in a big joint family, with uncles and their families. When stressed, mother used to beat her. Her father was a businessman and he never spent time with her. She had several cousins who did not show any love to her and she felt isolated and lonely. When she was 7 years, an older cousin abused her; she felt angry, but helpless. She had another trauma at that age; she lost a younger sister, who was delivered prematurely, whom she was eagerly waiting for. That also added to her anger. Three sessions of hypnotherapy were done in 10 days: age regression (she regressed back to age 7) and release of the childhood trauma and anger release in the adult were done. Her anger became under control and fear also reduced and she felt comfortable, relaxed and calm.

Many relationship issues originate from uncontrolled anger. Anger could be towards a particular person or a situation or a general behavioral disorder. The person may feel remorse afterwards and desire to change, but unable to do it. Then he/she seeks professional help. One to 3 sessions of hypnotherapy are found to produce the desired change in behavior. Hypnodrama is very effective in resolving anger towards individuals, while desensitization works well with general anger, even one session giving the desired effect (see chapter 7).

Fears and Phobias

Fears and phobias are a common reason why people seek professional help and an area where hypnotherapy has found tremendous success. When we are born, we have only two fears: fear of falling and fear of loud noise. All other fears are learned later and can be removed through hypnotherapy.

Fears usually have a known origin, and mostly start in the childhood, e.g. fear of dogs, fear of spiders, fear of ghosts, etc.

> Raghu, a 38 year old Mechanic, presented with a problem of unknown fear and tension. When he hears someone is sick, he feels sad, heart beats faster, then he becomes silent; the symptoms disappear after 10–15 minutes. Three sessions of hypnotherapy were done. After 2 sessions in which desensitization to feeling of fear was done, his fear reduced, but not completely gone. So in the 3rd session, after taking him into deep hypnosis, I asked him to go to the origin of his fear and he regressed back to an incident when he was 3 or 4 years old; while walking on the road with his grandmother, he was hit by a bicycle and fell down and became unconscious. After releasing the emotions of trauma from there, his fear left him and he became more confident.

In some cases even one session of hypnotherapy has been found to produce satisfactory results in overcoming fear.

> One of my clients, Vipin, 31 years, is an artist. He is unmarried and is living with his parents. He had an unhappy childhood, as his parents were always quarrelling, shouting at each other. He suffered from inferiority feeling, entertained negative thoughts and was afraid of interacting with people. One session of hypnotherapy removed his fear. Second session was done after 10 days in which suggestion was given to remove inferiority feeling, release negative thoughts and build confidence, and he became confident and positive.

In most cases, the person comes with more than one symptom, which they may not reveal in the beginning.

> Bhama, 69 years old, is a housewife. She had a surgery 4 years back, after which she developed fear that she may get isolated and left alone. In one session of hypnotherapy, she got rid of the fear. Then she said that she was experiencing constant sadness since she was eight years, when her mother died, and her father married again. One more session was done, and her sadness also left her.

Phobias are illogical fears without any known reason and usually seen in adults, e.g. fear of heights, fear of flying, fear of blood, fear of closed rooms (claustrophobia), etc. Sometimes it is difficult to know if it is a fear or phobia, then it is safe to treat it as phobia. In the case of Raghu, cited above, the client said he had a phobia, but it can be considered as fear, as there was a known reason, his accident on the road, which originated in the childhood, even though he could not remember it in the conscious state. Both fears and phobias can be removed completely by hypnotherapy – releasing the negative feelings and associations, installing a positive feeling like happiness, confidence, etc. and associating the new feeling with the triggering stimulus/situation. Once the subconscious mind accepts the new feeling, the person starts behaving on that basis.

Desensitization (see chapter 5) is a safe and effective method to treat phobias and adult fears; we ask them to bring up only the emotional feelings not the physical sensations and hence less traumatic to the client. Some common fears and phobias are listed in Table 2.

Table 2: Some Common Fears and Phobias

Fears	Phobias
Fear of animals (could also be phobia)	Acrophobia (Fear of heights)
Fear of dogs	Agoraphobia (fear of open spaces)
Fear of spiders	Claustrophobia (fear of closed spaces)
Fear of ghosts	
Fear of failure	Fear of animals
Fear of loss	Fear of crowds
Fear of pain	Fear of death and dying
Fear of public speaking	Fear of depths
Fear of rejection	Fear of flying (could also be fear)
Fear of responsibility	Hematophobia (fear of blood)
Fear of roads (could also be a phobia)	Hydrophobia (fear of water)
Fear of success	Fear of impending danger
Fear of strangers	Fear of contamination (mysophobia)
Fear of the unknown (could be phobia)	

Many phobias come from some traumatic experience that occurred in a past life and stored in the primitive memory. In such cases, past life regression therapy (explained in chapter 9) is used, in which the person is taken into very deep hypnosis, then regressed back to the original event that caused the phobia and healing done from there, which removes the present problem.

> I treated a client, a man of about 35 years, who was afraid of heights. He could not go up above the first floor of a building, he used to feel giddy and sad. He said he was scared of climbing on the boundary wall of his house, which is about 3 feet high. In the first session I helped him to release the fear through desensitization, but that gave only a short term benefit. In the second session, done after a month, under deep somnambulistic stage, I asked him to go to the origin of his fear. He went to an event in a past life; he is a young boy of about 8 years, living in a place with hillocks and small mountains around. He has some goats, and he takes them up a hill through a narrow path for grazing. While he is walking up, he slips down from the path, falls into the depth of the valley and dies. After that session his fear left him; later he informed me that he is very comfortable climbing up the boundary wall, and he went up to the 8th floor of his office building without any fear or discomfort. Reliving the incident in the past life helped him to release the trauma from its origin, resolving the problem in the present life

Anxiety

Anxiety is the fear about future and is a serious impediment in the normal functioning that severely affects the progress of a person. Many clients are confused about the actual problem; many a time what the client describes as fear or phobia turns out to be anxiety, which is identified through questioning during the pre-induction interview. Anxiety is treated as one treats a fear or phobia. Even one session has been found to produce spectacular results.

> Ashok, a 38 year old man, working in an Insurance company, felt severe anxiety when some relative goes to hospital; then he feels fear, palpitation of heart, and weakness in body. His kidneys are damaged, and he is waiting for kidney transplant, but is nervous about the operation and anxious about the outcome of transplantation. Three sessions of hypnotherapy were done and suggestions to reduce stress, release anxiety and remove fear of surgery were given. His anxiety was gone, and he felt relaxed and was looking forward to the operation.

Insomnia

Even though people approach me seeking help to remove insomnia, most of them are not aware that insomnia is not a problem by itself, but only a symptom indicative of some emotional or physical issue. Treating the underlying issue restores normal sleep, which is the approach used in hypnotherapy in treating insomnia.

> A 50 year old man running a shop, presented with insomnia and was taking medicines without which he was unable to sleep; probing questions revealed that he has lot of tension and insecurity feeling. He was also depressed. Three sessions of hypnotherapy were done, releasing the insecurity feeling, and suggestions to remove depression and build confidence were given, after which his tension and insecurity feeling left him and he started sleeping well without medicine.

Bereavement

The loss of some one dear is a very traumatic experience and can cause severe behavioral issues. Bereavement is generally associated with death. There are 5 stages of loss that everyone passes through till they come out of the trauma. These are denial, anger, depression, bargaining and resolution.

Denial is the first reaction, where the person refuses to accept that the loss has occurred. This is followed by anger, could be towards the person who has left or towards anyone who is available. Then comes depression, which can occur along with anger, the person going back and forth between these two stages. The fourth stage is bargaining, which can have a beneficial effect, leading to the final stage of resolution, where the person begins to put things in order and cope with the situation. Without intervention it can take even years to recover from the trauma and reach the stage of resolution.

Hypnotherapy helps the client to pass through the different stages to resolution, resulting in healing in a few sessions. So when a client with such an issue comes to me, the first thing I do is explain the different stages under conscious state and find out where he/she is at the current moment. Then under deep hypnosis, I take him/her through the different stages, one by one, in subsequent sessions till resolution is achieved. If the therapy starts at stage 1, it can take 5 to 7 sessions till complete resolution is achieved. The first three stages are the most difficult. Some people can get stuck in stage 1 or 2.

In some cases, after overcoming the first and second stages, the clients are able to resolve the remaining stages by themselves.

> A lady in her early 50s, a health professional, lost her only son aged 24 years due to cancer. Even though she was witness to the course of treatment to the final stage of death, she could not accept that her son is no more. She felt miserable, always crying, could not sleep properly, will wake up suddenly in the middle of the night and run out of the house, saying that her son is asking for some articles like spectacles, keys, etc. When she was brought to me, she had a peculiar expression on her face, a mixture of fear, anger and sadness, but she agreed for hypnotherapy. It took only two sessions of hypnotherapy, followed by one session of conscious counselling to bring her back to her normal routine and profession.

Similar reactions are encountered also in other relationships like divorce, break up from a love affair, or a grown up son/daughter leaving the family. The majority of the cases that have come to me are break up of love affair and the presenters are in the age range of 18 to 30. One of the partners is unable to come out of the trauma and goes into depression, even attempts suicide.

> A 23 year old final semester Engineering student was brought to me by her mother and elder brother. She was in love with a junior student, belonging to another religion. When the family knew about it, her father collapsed and was admitted in the hospital. She was feeling guilty and wanted to break off from her lover, as she also came to know that he was just flirting and had no intention of marriage. She felt cheated, became sad and depressed, but his memories were haunting her, and she was not able to recover from the trauma. Three sessions of hypnotherapy were done; first I desensitized her to the feeling of sadness and gave suggestion to overcome depression and build confidence. In the second and third sessions I also used a method called 'cord cutting' to emotionally disconnect with her former lover. She became cheerful, and free from the disturbing thoughts, and when she left my office she was laughing and joking with her mother and brother.

Here a few words about 'cord cutting' seem to be in place. When a person develops an affectionate relationship with another person, energy connections are established between the chakras of the two persons through which energy (emotions) is exchanged. This cord develops naturally between mother and child and exists from birth; in other relationships, including father and siblings, it develops later. In love relationships, under deep hypnosis it can be seen as a white cord between the solar chakras of the partners and the connection can be cut and severed, which will stop the energy exchange, freeing the person from the emotional attachment. This is a very effective method of releasing emotional trauma in divorces, breakdown of a romantic affair, and other damaging attachments like that between kidnapper and victim, between sexual abuser and victim, homosexual relationships, etc.

Relationship Issues

> Neeraja, a 34 year old IT professional approached me for help in straightening her family life. She has conflicts with her husband and feels angry, and distanced from him, sometimes even hatred towards husband. There was an ego clash between the two, which started after their engagement. After marriage, the conflict increased, she felt he does not give her freedom and impose restrictions on even decisions like what dresses she should wear. They have two children, elder boy and the younger a girl. After the birth of the son she went into post-partum depression, for which she was treated by a psychiatrist and took medicine for 3 years. Daughter was born after 7 years. Her son behaves in an irritating way and she feels tension. Two sessions of hypnotherapy were done with a gap of 2 weeks, in which suggestion to release tension was given and feelings of anger and hatred towards husband were released. She came after a week and said that she is comfortable and family relations are smooth; so she did not want another session.

Problems between couples are on the rise and divorce rates are increasing fast in the recent years. In most of the cases misunderstanding and lack of proper communication are found to be at the root of the problem. Arguments start on trivial, sometimes imagined, lapses that could have been sorted out through discussions; then communication becomes strained and even stops completely. The emotions get internalized and stored, accumulating the ill feeling, leading to break up of relationship, if not physically but emotionally. In such cases, if both the partners come with a genuine desire to resolve the problem, hypnotherapist can help them. Success is possible only if both the partners agree for change and are willing to participate in the treatment and committed to complete the treatment,

Incompatibility can also arise due to the difference in the basic characteristics of the persons involved. People can be divided into two general types – physical and emotional. Physical people are extroverts, expressive, emotional and physically reactive and right brain dominated, while emotional people are introverts, averse to physical expression and avoid being noticed by others and are left brain dominated. There is a general tendency among most people to view his/her behavior as right and in a relationship they want the other person to change according to his/her standards, whereas the partner does not find any reason why he/she should change. This creates misunderstanding leading to arguments, then lack of proper communication, aggravating the problem with time. When such people come to me, first I explain the different personal characteristics and how they can help themselves by accepting the other person as an individual with his/her own characteristics and preferences and find the best way to adopt a give-and-take attitude for the health and happiness of the family. Many a time this itself helps in resolving the issue. But in some cases, where either one or both partners are stubborn and insists that it is the other person who needs to change, it takes more effort and more sessions. If the damage is too far gone and beyond repair, and if the partners are not willing to accept the need for change, then it may be wise to leave them alone.

> A couple of years back a 61 year old man approached me for help to sort out a relationship issue. He said his wife is not giving him love and not allowing physical intimacy and he feels neglected and isolated in his family and sexually deprived. He was depressed, helpless and desperate. He said that he has been toiling for years to give a good life to his wife and two children, built a house for them with all physical comforts; so he could not give attention to his wife. Now that he is retired and stays at home, he expects his wife to spend time with him, catering to all his needs. But after the household works, she spends her time in devotional activities, reading religious books and doing worship in the Pooja room which irritates him. She does

not like to be with him, but is friendly with one of his cousins, a 34 year old man who gives attention to her and amuses her with stories and jokes; her husband feels neglected and side lined. I scheduled a session the next week and asked him to come with his wife. I talked to his wife separately and she said that she is doing what she used to do earlier for her husband and children. Turning to religious activities was her method of coping with her loneliness and frustration with her husband, who was busy earning money doing overtime work and neglecting her and not trying to know how she feels. Now that he is retired and at home and has time, he wants her to leave all those activities and spend time with him. But she no more enjoys his company or physical relations with him as he expects from her, for she does not love him but is doing her duties, cooking, washing and taking care of his health. When she came to his house as a young bride, he did not have time for her and she felt lonely, neglected and sad. She loves his younger cousin, although she knows that she cannot marry him, who gave her love and care when she needed it most. They grew closer in intimacy and her husband did not object or try to curb his visits. Her husband admitted that he could not give attention to her; since his father had died, as the eldest son, he had the responsibility of the family, educating the younger siblings, their marriage, mother's health, etc. But now that he has all the time for her, he expects his wife to understand his needs and change accordingly. Since his wife was not ready for that and he was not willing to consider changing himself, I could not do anything to help.

In traditional Indian families the head of the family decides everything, including what the other members are entitled to do, their responsibilities, how they should behave, and also the selection of marriage partners. In many families the rule is that the man decides and woman obeys, whether she likes it or not. As she is not allowed to express herself, she suppresses the feelings, which later leads to emotional and physical problems and creates fissures, sometimes irreparable damage to the relationship.

So in the first session I talk to both the partners and make a general assessment of the situation and then ask them if they are committed to saving the relationship and ready for the change that may be required on each one's part and to complete the treatment. I continue only if the answers of both the partners are in the affirmative. But many a time after starting the treatment their personal ego comes in the way and one of them discontinues, then the therapist cannot do anything to help. But with those couples who are committed to repair the damage, hypnotherapy has been successful. Dissatisfaction with sexual life has been found to create problems between couples. Many a time the cause lies in the childhood or in a past life.

> A 25 year old lady was brought to me by her husband. They are married for 5 years and have a 3 year old son. But the wife is afraid of sex, even averse to physical intimacy and looked for excuses to avoid sex. Two sessions of hypnotherapy were able to resolve the issue. As I was taking her into deep hypnosis, she suddenly said 'fire' in Hindi, which is not her familiar language. She had regressed back to a life in Northern India. She saw herself as a 5 year old girl, playing outside her mud house in a village. A group of dacoits come on horseback and the villagers rush inside their houses and close the doors and the child is left outside. The dacoits burn the houses, killing all the people. As they are leaving the area, one of them sees the child and carries her with him. The child grows up in the dacoit's camp, doing the household works like cooking, cleaning, etc. As she attains puberty, they start using her for their sexual pleasures. At the age of 35, she is sick with venereal diseases and is abandoned to die with no one, except her 15 year old son near her. The fear of sexual intimacy in the current life came from the memory of the traumatic experiences, carried forward from that life. After that session, her fear and aversion to sex disappeared.

Relationship issues are also seen between parent and son/daughter, where the attachment is too strong, On separation due to marriage of the daughter or when son/daughter settles in another city/country, abandoning the old parents. In such cases, suggestion to accept and adjust to the new situation in the absence of viable alternatives, given under hypnosis, can help the client to look at the situation in a new and positive perspective, leading to catharsis.

In breakdown of love affair and divorce, most of the clients who sought my help or brought to me by parents are women between 19 and 35. Since the relationship has ended, with no hope of retrieval, my attempt is to release the trauma and bring the person back to normal life and activities, with an optimistic mindset.

Some cases of older people who got into an extra-marital affair and want to detach from the person have been treated successfully through cord cutting.

A temple priest, 55 years, married and living with wife and a grown up son, developed an attachment with a younger woman 3 months back. He started helping her with money, which led to frequent phone calls, then they had physical relations and he started neglecting his wife. This affected his family life and he wanted to stop that extra-marital relationship but was not able to do it. That is when his son brought him to me. I did cord cutting (two sessions) and he left the relationship and felt free and comfortable. One more session was done, in which suggestion to release negative feelings (he was feeling guilty and ashamed) and fill in feeling of happiness was given. Three sessions were enough to resolve the problem and restore harmony in their life.

Improving Performance Skills in Sports and Other Areas

A 22 year old graduate student and National level shooting champion, living in Mumbai, came for hypnotherapy. She does well in practice sessions, but in the matches, she was not able to come up to the expected level of excellence that she used to get earlier. She has been in the shooting team since she was 15 years. She has a good coach, a former Olympian, best facilities and parents were supportive, but she was not able to put her full form into it. She lost interest in the sport and often skipped the practice sessions. She said that she has no passion or love for it.

When she was in the 10th standard, they had shifted from Jaipur to Pune. It was her parents' decision, although she did not want to go to Pune. Parents thought it will be best for her career, as there are better facilities in Pune and after 5 years they moved to Mumbai. She felt that her parents are overprotective and decided everything for her and did not allow her to do anything on her own. So there used to be quarrels between her and her parents. She feels locked in, frustrated, angry, stressed, anxious. She wants to cry, but she is not able to cry. There was lot of anger towards parents; she felt they are one team, and she is another team. Four sessions of hypnotherapy were done; anger towards parents (hypnodrama) was released in the first session and she was able to talk to her mother without anger, she felt more loving towards father and mother. The next 3 sessions were used to remove anxiety about her sports performance with guided imagery to improve the shooting performance and suggestion for motivation to practice regularly with concentration, and she became more positive and enthusiastic about the sport.

A 37 year old male, screen actor, came for help in improving his screen performance. He had anxiety while facing the camera which affected his acting career. Four sessions of hypnotherapy were done. In the first session, suggestions to remove anxiety and build confidence were given; this was followed by guided imagery – from waiting for the vehicle to go to the location, standing in front of the camera, feeling relaxed and confident, Director giving the signal to start, he performing with confidence, saying the dialogues correctly, with proper emotions, etc. to the Director saying 'cut' and okaying the scene, he going back to his seat, feeling happy. Suggestion to build confidence and guided imagery were repeated during the next 2 sessions and guided imagery was repeated in the last session, and he became comfortable in front of the camera.

Reasons for inability to perform well in their field of interest vary with different people and the therapist helps to remove the handicap and bring out the talent to its maximum extent. It should be remembered that in such cases the therapist is not creating something new, but only helps in bringing out what is already there in the person and improving on it. So if a person does not have the basic talent, therapist will not be able to help. I am pointing this out because some parents approach me with requests to install new talents in their children; for example, a mother wanted to become a dancer, but due to the circumstances she could not achieve her ambition. So she wanted her daughter to become a dancer, even though the child did not have the talent or desire to learn dance, and sought my help to create interest for dance in the child through hypnotherapy. Similarly, some parents have approached me with the expectation that hypnotherapy can increase the comprehensive level of children with severe mental retardation. I explain to them that this is a condition that the soul of the child has voluntarily created to fulfil the purpose of its incarnation, so they have to accept it. We do not try to change something that is inborn, but it is possible to change what is acquired after birth.

In some cases, the origin of the problem may lie in a past life, where past life regression therapy (see chapter 9) is found to be effective in overcoming the handicap and improving the efficiency in performance.

A lady in her early 50s was brought to me by her son. She was a music teacher, also giving private lessons in music at home, but for the last 2 or 3 years she was not able to sing. When she tried to sing, she felt some constriction in the throat, her vocal cords getting tight and the tune did not come out; otherwise she was able to speak fluently. There was no reason she could think of which could have caused the problem. I took her into very deep hypnosis and guided her through suggestion to the origin of her problem. She regressed back to a life about 150 years ago, as a woman living in Kerala. She is an expert vocalist and is appointed by the king to teach music to the princess. One day when she was with the princess, she saw a male servant in the king's court stealing something. She reported it to the queen, and he was removed from the job. But that man wanted to take revenge on the music teacher. One day when she was alone in the room, he came and said that because of her throat she was enjoying the favor of the royal family and complained to them, and she is not going to do it anymore. He caught hold of her throat and strangled her and she died. After reliving the experience and disconnecting with that life, she regained her ability to sing and started teaching music.

Stammering

Deepak, a 24 year old man wanted help to overcome his problem with speech. He had stammering from the time he started speaking at the age of 2 or so. He was so conscious of it that he was unable to speak to strangers or in front of a group. He was well educated and academically qualified but lost several job opportunities because he refrained from attending the interview. His sister said that there are two interviews next month, which he should not miss, but he is reluctant to attend them. He attended 3 sessions of hypnotherapy, in which, under deep hypnosis, I gave suggestions to desensitize to the specific situations that caused stammering and build confidence and self-esteem. In the second and third sessions, in addition to the suggestions, I also did a guided imagery of his attending the interview with confidence, taking him through the whole process, ending up with his selection for the job and returning home feeling happy and proud of his achievement. We scheduled a 4th session, but he did not turn up. Later that day his mother phoned to tell that he had gone to attend a job interview. He performed well in the interview and was selected. His stammering was more controlled, but not totally gone.

Some stammering, especially those developed later in childhood or adult life, are easier to remove, but in some cases the reasons may be deeper rooted. It may take several sessions to achieve the full effect at the physical level. Even in cases where the stammering may not be stopped completely, the person can be made confident and ready to face the situation boldly and effectively through suggestions, as seen in the above case. Stammering in some cases is found to have its origin in a childhood experience.

A 30 year old man, a science graduate, working as a Technician, came to me for help in stopping stammering. His speech was normal while speaking to his friends. But when talking to strangers, asking for direction on the road, etc. he gets stuck at certain words. Then he feels fear and tension, and his lips tremble. His childhood was happy and there was no problem with his speech. Stammering started when he was in the 10th std. His teacher asked a question in the class. While trying to answer the words did not come and he felt fear and shame. After that in the higher classes and in College (he is a graduate in Physics) he had stammering when speaking in front of people, reading in the class, or when angry. He took Ayurveda medicines for 4–5 months but did not get any benefit. Four sessions of hypnotherapy were done. After 2 sessions in which feelings of fear and tension were released, he was more confident and his speech improved, but he still felt difficulty in pronouncing some words while speaking to strangers. In the next session, after taking him into a deep somnambulistic stage, he was led through suggestions to the origin of the cause of his problem and he regressed back to an event when he was in the 3rd standard. He is in the class. The teacher is asking him to recite a poem and he is stammering; other students are laughing; he feels sad and weak in body. After releasing the disturbing feelings experienced by the child there, desensitization of the adult to the emotional feelings associated with stammering was done and the space filled with feeling of confidence. His problem reduced considerably, he felt difficulty only with one or two words and became confident of speaking to even strangers. He did not come for further session.

Study Problems

Mostly children studying in classes 10 to 12 are brought by parents before the examinations, the commonly reported problems being lack of concentration and poor time management. Young people studying in the Professional courses and those appearing for competitive examinations and entrance tests also seek my help. Two to four sessions of hypnotherapy, in which suggestion to increase concentration and time management given under medium trance are found to produce the desired change. But some youngsters who seek help in improving study habits also exhibit other problems like low confidence, anxiety and fear. They may need more sessions to achieve the full effect.

Viraj, a 19 year old Engineering student, was brought to me by his parents, with the complaint that he was not able to concentrate on studies. He wanted to become an Automobile Engineer. He did not have any regular study pattern. His father was overcritical, and never appreciated anything his son does or encouraged him.

I asked Viraj to make a timetable for his daily studies; under hypnosis I gave a suggestion to improve study habits, including the time table, followed by suggestion to increase concentration. After two sessions he started studying with more concentration. One more session was done to reinforce the effect and that resolved his study problem. I also counselled his father to be more understanding and appreciate when he does something positive.

More cases are discussed in chapter 14.

Addictions and Harmful Habits

Amar, a businessman in his early 50s, sought my help in stopping alcohol drinking. He was drinking daily in the evenings, which his wife, a government employee, objected to, and there were regular quarrels over this between them. Their only son, studying for a Professional degree, also found his father's addiction stressful, disturbing the peace of the family, and got irritated and angry. Amar came voluntarily to me with the desire to stop drinking. After 3 sessions of hypnotherapy, in which suggestion to stop drinking and develop aversion towards alcohol was given and he stopped drinking completely. Then he said he has the habit of smoking cigarettes which he wants to quit. He had tried to stop smoking a few times but could not succeed. So during the next 3–4 sessions, suggestion to quit smoking, emphasizing the benefits of being a non-smoker was given, followed by guided imagery to reinforce the new behavior in different scenarios where he is refusing the offer of cigarettes while his friends are smoking and he feels proud that he is a non-smoker. He left the habit forever. With his quitting alcohol and smoking, the atmosphere in the family became peaceful and he was spending more time with his wife and son and enjoying it. Then he wanted to stop chewing tobacco, which was achieved in 2 sessions. Now, about 6 years after his last session with me, he said he does not find alcohol tempting even when he sits in a bar with friends who drink and he chooses plain water or some soft drinks; he does not use cigarettes or any form of tobacco. His family life has become peaceful and happy.

Alcoholism is the most common addiction for which people seek my help. So far only male clients have come to me, the majority of them in the age range of 30 to 65 years. In many cases clients who drink alcohol also have the habit of smoking or using other tobacco products. In India, especially the middle class families, generally females are not found to fall into alcohol addiction or smoking, but tobacco chewing is not uncommon, especially in the older people; but they do not want to leave the habit although mouth cancer incidence is high among both males and females, especially in some parts of rural India where tobacco chewing is widespread.

Even though hypnotherapy is very effective in permanently eliminating addictions success is possible only if the client wants it and willing to stick to the therapy to completion. So first I ask the client if it is his desire to stop it or he is doing it for someone else's sake. Only if the person volunteers for it I start the therapy. But sometimes, under pressure from the family or because the doctor asked him, a client may say that it is his desire and is willing to complete the treatment, then discontinues after a couple of sessions.

> A 65 year old man, running a grocery store, was brought to me by his wife and grown up son. After closing his shop in the evening, on his way home, he used to go to a local pub and drink daily. His family wanted him to stop drinking as it was affecting his health. But he was not ready for it. When his wife called me to book an appointment, I had told her that hypnotherapy will succeed only if he wants to stop it. So the family doctored him to say that he has come willingly. After two sessions, without any change in his habit, he confessed that he cannot live without 2 pegs a day and he had agreed for therapy under pressure from the family. I told the family about the futility of the treatment, which was discontinued.

If the client comes with a firm resolve to quit the habit, even a couple of sessions has been found to yield incredible outcome.

> A young man of 40, single, and living with his widowed mother was addicted to alcohol and smoking. His mother was very worried about his future and under lot of tension. He wanted to stop drinking and smoking for the sake of his mother. He also had diabetes. After four sessions he was totally free from both alcohol and cigarettes and his mother became tension free and happy. One more session was done to reinforce the effect and he never needed any further treatment for these issues. His blood sugar also came under control.

The following case shows that with a firm resolve on the part of the client, even one session of hypnotherapy can produce spectacular changes.

> A middle aged Legal Adviser, a chain smoker, smoking 40–50 cigarettes a day, approached me for help to quit smoking. In such cases, usually I suggest a long treatment, lasting 5–6 sessions in 6 or 7 weeks, with a gradual reduction in the number of cigarettes and finally quitting completely. He said that it is not going to work as he does not have the patience. So we opted for a short treatment, even though I was not optimistic. After the first session on an afternoon, his second session was scheduled for the next morning, the gap between the sessions being about 20 hours. When he came for the second session, he surprised me with the statement that since he went home after the first session he had not smoked even a single cigarette and he was feeling fine. Two more sessions were done to reinforce the effect and to remove the urge for smoking.

A possible side effect of such a drastic change is the tendency for the person to put on weight, which can be controlled by regular practice of yoga and other exercises. The advantage of hypnotherapy is that it takes care of the withdrawal syndromes, without the client becoming aware of them, so the recovery is smooth and without discomfort.

Hypnotherapy can also help in de-addiction of drug abusers. But a major obstacle in treating drug addicts is that they come after being in de-addiction centers and they have fear of the severe withdrawal syndromes. Most of the time the clients do not come on their own but are brought by the parents or spouse and they may not get involved in the treatment, which is essential for the treatment to be effective. Even if the client comes willingly, they are not able to stick to the treatment schedule and complete it, and they tell a lot of lies. They may say it is not a habit and they can stop any time they want, or a friend gave it to them, and they consumed it without knowing it, etc. The family also needs to be patient and give emotional support to the client, considering him/her as a sick person who needs help to recover. The few people, young men in the range of 18–25 years, who were brought to me did not come back after the first session. To some extent, the parents are also responsible for this, as it is considered to be a social stigma on the family and they fear what others will say if they come to know that someone in their family is a drug addict. But they should realize it is the future of their child and they have to stand with him/her, have patience, understanding the mental condition of the person and assuring emotional support and security.

Chapter Twelve
Clinical Applications

Hypnotherapy has found a place, as an individual modality or as an adjuvant to other treatments, in several clinically diagnosed diseases. Medical centers like the Mayo Clinic in USA are using hypnotherapy as an alternative and complementary treatment. In India, people consider hypnotherapy as a last resort when all other options are exhausted, and the conventional treatments fail to give the desired result.

Some of the clinical problems for which people usually seek my help are discussed below.

Pain Relief

This is perhaps the most accepted use of hypnotherapy in the clinical settings. It can be used effectively in all types of pain, acute and chronic.

> One of my first clients was a 77 year old man, retired from Central Government service in 1991, who was suffering from pain in both knees since the last about 10 years. He was taking homeopathy medicines and also doing some oil massage, but the pain continued. I had recently started my practice when he approached me. I explained hypnotherapy to him and told that it does not use medicines and works at the mind level. As he is religious and believes in the power of mind, he wanted to try it and was receptive to the suggestions. As he had difficulty in sitting continuously, he was made to lie down; hypnosis was induced by progressive relaxation and deepened further to somnambulistic stage. Then pain relief was done by imagining the pain as an object and eliminating the pain by destroying that object, taking it as the symbol of the pain. On waking

up he felt relief from pain. A second session was done the next week, repeating the same process of creating a symbol of the pain and eliminating it. He got complete relief from his knee pain with two sessions. Now he is over 90 years; even though he has other age related problems like loss of hearing and some dementia, his knee pain has not returned.

Pain is a prominent and essential symptom in many diseases, from a mild headache associated with common cold, to the intense sensation felt in more serious conditions like migraines, fractures, burns, surgery, etc. Hence a major application of hypnotherapy in clinical conditions could be giving relief from pain. According to hypnotherapy concept, pain originates in the mind before it is sensed by the brain; therefore, it can be treated successfully by hypnotherapy. There is ample empirical evidence to support and confirm this. This is recognized by the World Health Organization (WHO).

There are several published reports supporting the analgesic effect of hypnotherapy in clinical contexts. Posthypnotic suggestions are found to give lasting relief from pain associated with arthritis, back injury, cancers, sciatica, spinal injury, etc.

Arthritis and other Joint Pains

Arthritis is a common affliction reported by people above 50, for which a permanent remedy is not found in the conventional therapies. Medicines, massages and physical exercises are prescribed which continue throughout life. A few sessions of hypnotherapy are found to relieve the pain and maintain a comfortable condition.

Roopa, a 61 year old housewife, diagnosed with rheumatoid arthritis, was under Allopathic treatment for 20 years. When she came to me, she had severe pain on the underside of both feet and in the toes; her toes were getting numb and bending to one side, which she could not straighten. There was pain in the ankles also and it was difficult for her to walk without support. Four sessions of hypnotherapy were done. After 3 sessions, she got complete relief from the pain and the toes became straight and she started walking without help. Suggestion for a general healing was given in the 4th session. After one year she was free of the pain and had stopped the use of analgesics.

Pain is a natural response, a signal coming from the subconscious mind for seeking attention of the conscious mind to that part for remedial action. So I do not recommend removing it completely in arthritis, fractures, etc., because the client may become careless in taking the necessary precautions and overuse the part, which can have a counter-effect.

> A housewife, in her early 60s, had bone degeneration and pain in knee joints of both legs. Before treating for knee pain I had cautioned her not to stand continuously for long or overuse the legs. Hypnotherapy gave relief from pain, but after 6 months she came back with the complaint that the pain has returned. When I asked her what she did to bring back the pain, she said that as her daughter and grandchildren were visiting, she cooked their favorite dishes standing for many hours in the kitchen. Again I helped her in relieving the pain, this time leaving behind about 10% as a caution. After that she did not come back with the same complaint.

Back Pain

This is another common complaint that brings people to me.

> Manju, 45years, a kitchen help in a health care center, was referred to me. She was suffering from pain in the middle back for the last few years and was using a corset. She was ready for hypnosis and easily went deep. Three sessions of hypnotherapy were done; I used a technique of miniaturization and made her enter the body and view the problem *in situ* and heal from there. The pain was gone, and she became comfortable without the corset.

Miniaturization is a useful technique for healing physical problems. It is done under very deep somnambulistic stage of hypnosis. In this state, anything is possible; whatever the subconscious mind imagines becomes the fact. The consciousness of the person is asked to come out of the body and reduce itself to a miniature size, then enter the body. Then it is guided to the problem area/organ and asked to describe the condition. The person will describe the problem as he/she perceives it. It need not be an anatomical description. One can even talk to the cells and find out why they have created the problem and how it can be corrected and follow what they say. Each cell has its own intelligence and consciousness and there is always a purpose for bringing about the condition; it is their own creation and, therefore, can be undone. Once the change is made, it becomes the reality for the mind. The mind then makes the body change accordingly, resulting in healing.

A sedentary lifestyle, sitting in the same position for long and lack of exercise are causing back pain and posture complaints in many young and middle aged people, especially those working in the IT field. In such cases after the pain relief is done, I also suggest regular Yoga practice and exercises to maintain the health.

> Rajan, a 37 year old IT professional, working in an international company approached me with severe back pain. He had consulted an Orthopedic surgeon who suggested an operation to correct a vertebral injury, which, he said, was causing the pain. Rajan was afraid of the operation and while searching the internet for an alternative, he came to know of hypnotherapy and called me and fixed an appointment. He was not able to sit for long, so hypnotherapy was done in the lying position. He went easily into deep hypnosis. Using the miniaturization suggestion, I guided him to the area of the injury, and he described the problem as a vertebra broken into pieces; he repaired it using cement and mortar. Suggestion was also given to reduce pain and accelerate healing. After one session he was able to sit comfortably in the chair. After the second session, in which under deep hypnosis he visualized the vertebra completely healed and healthy, his back felt comfortable. He did not come again or give a feedback. But after a few months he referred a friend to me, who said Rajan did not have the operation, and is healthy, even playing cricket.

In some cases, even though the person presents with back pain, that may not be the only problem. Therefore, more than one technique has to be employed, addressing each problem separately till complete relief is obtained.

> Soumini, a 58 year old woman, was brought to me with the complaint of pain in the middle back, hips, neck, knees and right hand. She was not able to lift even small things or could not tie her Sari, as she felt intense pain with the movements. She could also not sleep well. She felt mental stress and sadness and anger towards her husband. Five sessions of hypnotherapy were done. In the first

2 sessions, pain release was done, taking pain as an object and reducing it to a comfortable minimum and she got relief from her back pain. During the next sessions, stress reduction, desensitization to sadness and release of anger towards husband (hypnodrama) were done. She became comfortable and was satisfied with her health.

Menstrual Pain

This is a complaint that brings many young women for therapy. The pain is very intense, sometimes accompanied with headache, vomiting, even fainting in some cases. It affects all their activities and upsets the routine. Hypnotherapy has been able to give permanent relief from menstrual pain and the accompanying discomforts.

Raji, a 26 year old Music student was brought to me by her mother. At the onset of her monthly periods she experienced intense pain in the abdominal area, which lasted one full day, then subsided. She felt weak in body and could not get up from bed; sometimes the pain was accompanied by nausea and vomiting. Only two sessions of hypnotherapy with a gap of 4 days gave complete relief from her problem.

Surabhi, a 23 year old Engineering student, came with severe pain associated with menstruation. The pain was so intense and debilitating that she had to take leave for the day. Her problem was resolved in two sessions of hypnotherapy and pain was totally eliminated. In the 8 years after the therapy she never had the pain again.

Even older clients in their 30s, who suffered from intense menstrual pain and approached me for help, have been treated successfully; in most cases 2–3 sessions gave complete relief.

Cancer Pain

In very advanced cases of cancer, where the disease has spread to different organs, it may not be possible to get complete healing, but the quality of life can be improved by reducing pain, and releasing negative emotions and bringing acceptance of the condition. The National Cancer Institute, USA, has recommended the use of hypnotherapy for pain control in cancer patients. In terminal cancer patients on morphine and in those under palliative care, hypnotherapy is found to produce lasting relief from pain, reducing or eliminating the use of chemical analgesics.

The cases of the elderly lady with recurrence of anal cancer and that of the young boy whose cancer had spread to bone, reported in chapter 1, show how hypnotherapy can give relief and improve quality of life even in very advanced stages of cancer. One of the cases is described briefly below, for your ready reference.

> A 72 year old housewife was suffering from cancer in the colon, the lower part of her intestine, and had undergone surgery, radiotherapy, etc. Now the disease had come back, spread to other parts. There was a growth in the anal region which caused intense pain while passing stool. Pain killers, even morphine was not able to relieve the pain when she was referred to me. Even though she felt hungry, she was afraid of taking food thinking of the pain. She had difficulty in passing urine also. She agreed for hypnotherapy.
>
> Under deep hypnosis she imagined the pain as many pins sticking into the organ. Pain was relieved by pulling out those pins. It took three sessions to bring noticeable reduction in the pain. After the 4th session she embraced me and, with tears in her eyes, said (in her language, Hindi) 'daughter, you have taken away my agony.' It was a moment I cherish and thank God for making me choose this path. As the doctors had predicted, she died in a few months; but she was comfortable while passing stool and urine and eating normal food and sleeping well as long as she lived.

Migraine

It was in December 2007 that Karthik, a 47 year old man, an Assistant Manager in a private company, presented with a history of more than 20 years of frequent migraine attacks. In the beginning it was once in 2 or 3 months, the frequency gradually increased with time. Now, for the last 2–3 years he is getting migraine 1–2 times every month. Medicines gave only temporary relief. The headache was very intense, accompanied by aversion to light and sound, nausea, giddiness, and sometimes fainting.

The reason he came to me was because a month back, on his way to the bank to deposit money in the Company account, he got severe headache and fainted. Some people reached him to the nearby hospital, but when he came to his senses, he found the entire money missing. As he did not know how he reached the hospital or who were near him when he fainted, it was not possible to trace the money. The Company asked him to return the money in a short time. Since his migraine was at the root of his financial loss, he was looking for a permanent cure and approached me.

His was a small family with wife and one son, and life was comfortable. He could not give any particular reason for his migraine attacks. On questioning him in detail he admitted that he was stressed. I explained hypnotherapy and how it helps in de-stressing and relieving pain, and he agreed to be hypnotised. He went into deep somnambulistic stage easily. Suggestion for stress reduction, followed by desensitization to stressful situations was done. On waking up he felt relaxed and happy. A second session was done after 2 days, in which suggestions were given under deep hypnosis for stress reduction and building confidence. This was repeated after 2 days. Three sessions were done in total and his migraine disappeared. I met him in January 2020 at a function and he said that he never experienced migraine headaches after that treatment done 12 years back.

Migraines are among the most debilitating headaches, which still have not found a lasting remedy in the conventional therapies. It is a psychosomatic disorder, also called vascular headache, because it is thought to be caused by constriction of blood vessels, restricting blood flow to the brain. Generally, migraine does not have a physical basis. It can start suddenly without any obvious reason, usually on one side of the head and then spreads and can extend to the entire head in some cases. Pain is very intense and may last from twenty four to forty eight hours or more. The person may feel strong aversion to light, sound, smell, and even to presence of people around. Severe pain can lead to giddiness, sometimes nausea, vomiting, even fainting.

Triggers vary from person to person and include climatic conditions like intense heat or cold, physiological factors like hormonal changes associated with menstruation and menopause, hunger, sleep deprivation, or intense emotions like anger, grief, emotional outbursts, etc. Two to 4 sessions of hypnotherapy are found to give permanent relief from most migraines.

A 59 year old lady, a Bank Manager, was suffering from migraine for more than 20 years. She had lot of tension and anxiety, which triggered the headache. Three sessions of hypnotherapy were done; in the first session suggestions to release tension and anxiety were given and two sessions were devoted to address migraine, which gave relief from her problem.

Alka, in her early 30s, an IT professional, working in a private company, used to get severe migraine, especially before menstrual period. It was so severe that she had to take leave from office. Three sessions of hypnotherapy got rid of her problem and the occurrence of migraine stopped completely.

Vani, a 49 year old lady doctor was suffering from migraine since her school days. She used to get severe headache if she skips a meal, goes out in the hot sun, or her sleep was disturbed and lasted up to a week. She was irritated by bright light, felt weak in body and wanted to just lie down. Three sessions of hypnotherapy, in which desensitization to triggering situations and confidence building were done, gave complete relief. Now it is about 7 years after the therapy, and she has never experienced migraine during this period.

Depression

"Please doctor, I want to stop the medicines. Please help me." This was a 68 year old housewife, a post graduate degree holder, with a medical history of depression for the last 20 years.

Depression is not a single disease, but a complex of symptoms, both emotional and physical. Symptoms may vary from person to person. Major depression, also known as unipolar depression or major depression disorder (MDD), is characterized by persistent feeling of sadness, or a general lack of interest in daily activities. People exhibit different behavioral changes and reactions to how one feels. The main symptoms are given below; any five of these symptoms, occurring consistently and continuously for a period of 14 days or more can be considered major depression.

1. Negative thinking and inability to see positive solutions to problems
2. Feeling of worthlessness, and despair

3. Persistent low mood
4. Anxiety, lack of control on emotions
5. Hopelessness and helplessness, guilt feeling
6. Excessive crying or sadness
7. Restlessness, agitation and irritation
8. Inability to focus
9. Anger outbursts, especially against persons close to them
10. Lack of interest in daily routines and withdrawal from regular activities
11. Social isolation
12. Fatigue and lethargy
13. Insomnia or oversleep
14. Loss or gain of weight
15. Lack of appetite or overeating
16. Suicidal thoughts and/or attempts

Causes vary from person to person; failure in examination, business loss, loss of job, death or separation of a loved one, divorce, break up of relationship, chronic health problems or diseases like cancer, AIDS, constant negative thoughts, etc. can lead to depression.

Hypnotic approach to depression is based on how the client perceives the problem at the physical and emotional levels. Treatment can take many sessions, addressing each issue separately.

> The 68 year old housewife, mentioned above, was brought to me by her husband, a medical doctor. They have 3 children, all in the medical field, living abroad. She is a family person, very caring and concerned about the children. She was socially active, helpful and sensitive to others' problems. Her first episode of depression was in 1972, which disappeared after one month treatment with medicine. She was problem-free for more than 10 years, active, cheerful, easily mingling with people, enjoying family life and social activities.

Then she had a severe attack of depression, which was controlled by psychiatric treatment for 6 months, and treatment was stopped. The problem recurred after five years and needed medication. Initially the medicines gave relief from the symptoms, and she remained symptom-free for a couple of years, gradually the frequency increased. When she was brought to me in January 2009, she was on continuous medication for the last two years, but not able to lead a normal life. Now the benefit of medicines lasted 1–2 days only.

Most of the time she remained gloomy, suddenly crying or getting angry without reason, not taking interest in daily routines, does not like to talk to anyone, not interested in food, and unable to sleep. She did not have any other major health problems like diabetes, hypertension or cardiac problems, seen in women of that age group. The first thing she told on seeing me was that she wants to be free from medication, as the medicines were making her drowsy, lethargic, and unable to do even routine activities. I briefly explained hypnotherapy to her and her husband and told them that the treatment can take several sessions and the medicines can be reduced gradually with the permission of the psychiatrist and they agreed. Different emotional issues like sadness, anger, fear, anxiety, and mental and physical problems like negative thoughts, insomnia, fatigue, lethargy, etc. were addressed. After six sessions of hypnotherapy between 5th January and 30th January 2009, she returned to normal life and was able to gradually cut down on her medicines and stop them after 6 months. She remained that way for almost two years. Again she was brought to me on 30th October 2010, symptoms being sudden outbursts of anger, disturbed sleep, uneasiness, and lethargy. Five sessions of hypnotherapy were done in two months, which gave her complete relief from her symptoms. She was leading a normal life, involved in household activities, participating in family and social functions, cheerful and happy.

Again, after 4 years, in October 2014, she came with burning sensation in the feet and symptoms like fatigue and lethargy, lack of appetite and reduced interest in daily activities, insomnia and sadness, which were milder than earlier. Eight sessions of hypnotherapy were done during the next 10 months and she returned to normal life and activities; as of now, she is doing fine.

Another case of major depression, a 48 year old woman, married, with no children, was brought to me by her husband in November 2009. Her problem had started as a teenager, and once she had tried to commit suicide. She was shown to a Psychiatrist, who gave medicines that brought some relief. Then she was married and started living with her husband and parents-in-law. She had problems in adjusting with the husband's family. She was quarrelsome, fighting with her husband even for small things, always gloomy, not interested in mingling with people, unable to sleep, and showed suicidal tendencies. They consulted a psychiatrist who diagnosed depression and prescribed medicines. Since then she was being treated for depression and for about 20 years now she has been taking medicines, the doses were increased several times during this period. When I saw her, she was drowsy and sleepy most of the time, unable to respond to people, socially isolated, non-communicative, easily prone to tears or bursts of anger, with reduced and disturbed sleep in the night. She was in tears when she approached me, very sad and disappointed that she is not able to be a good wife and fulfil the duties to her husband and other family members.

She was ready for hypnosis. The treatment started on 30th November 2009. The whole treatment took 16 sessions, spread over a period of about 15 months. The first 2–3 sessions were devoted to relaxation and building confidence. She became calmer and in control but was not able to sleep well. She also experienced some unknown fear when alone. During the next few sessions, suggestions were given to build a positive attitude towards life in general, and to release anger and fear, and to improve sleep. Her condition improved considerably, and she was able to reduce the medicines. She started taking interest in household work, was feeling more relaxed, drowsiness had gone, and she was sleeping better during the night.

But after a few months, she came back with a recurrence of her symptoms. Her fear had returned, along with a feeling of helplessness and extreme sadness. So we decided on regression, as I felt there could be some past traumatic experience behind her problem. After taking her into very deep hypnosis, I asked her to go to the origin of her fear and feeling of helplessness. It took four sessions to reach the origin. In the first two sessions, she went to early childhood, where mother had left her alone in the room and she was afraid and felt helpless. When explaining the experience she showed extreme emotion on her face and trembling and choking. Releasing the childhood trauma gave relief from her symptoms, but not complete recovery. So past life regression was done; two sessions were needed to get the details. She saw herself as a 14 year old girl, working as a household help. It is a small village, year 1960 (Client was born in 1961). She is drawing water from the common well and slips down and falls into the well and gets drowned. She is afraid and feeling helpless, as there is nobody nearby who can hear her and help, and she dies. While narrating the experience, she showed the same kind of reactions, emotions on face and trembling, as those described earlier in cognitive state. With that session her fear and feeling of helplessness totally disappeared. After one more session, to increase confidence and improve her social interaction, the treatment was stopped. Her last hypnotherapy session was on February 7, 2011. Since then she is leading a normal life. Her medicines are almost completely stopped. She is happy, actively engaged in household works, has good interactions with husband's family members, taking part in family functions, sleeping well without help of medicine, and revived interest in reading and religious activities.

In the other depression patients who sought my help, the condition was less advanced and was resolved in fewer sessions.

Hema, a 29 year old woman, with two sons aged 10 and 8 years, was on anti-depressants for the last 3 years. She was married at 17 and was living with her husband and his parents. Her husband is an alcoholic and is abusive. Her mother-in-law also used to beat her. In the beginning, she used to silently suffer everything. Three years back when her mother-in-law beat her, she retaliated violently. She was taken to a psychiatrist and was hospitalized for 2 weeks. Her parents brought her back to their house, now she is staying separately near her parents' house and her mother is looking after her. Her children are adopted by an institution and being educated and taken care of by them. She was worried about the children and afraid that her husband will take them away. She was always sitting in the room and crying, showing no interest in even daily routines like taking bath, changing dress or eating, not talking to anyone, even to parents. After 3 sessions of hypnotherapy in which suggestions were given to release sad feelings and motivating her to take care of herself and get involved in household work, she became cheerful, smiling more often, and started taking interest in cooking, cleaning, taking bath daily, and watching TV. She visited her children and was happy that they are safe and taken care of. One more session was done to build confidence and she became happy and started interacting with family members and neighbors.

Different people suffering from depression exhibit different symptoms. In the above case sadness was the major symptom. Other prominent emotions include anxiety, fear, anger, and/or guilt, diffidence, inferiority and insecurity feeling. Physical symptoms like fatigue, body pain, headache, loss of energy, etc. are also seen.

Lalit, a 34 year old office clerk, was on anti-depressants for about 10 years when he approached me. He was tense and sad and had fear, anger and insecurity feeling. He was low in confidence and entertained inferiority feeling. He always felt tired and low in energy. In the first 3 sessions of hypnotherapy, stress reduction and release of sadness, fear and anger were done. Two more sessions were done to increase confidence and self-esteem and he stopped the medicines.

Some depressions can have their origin in a past life.

Ashish, a 22 year old student was suffering from extreme sadness, depression and suicidal thoughts for one and half years when he came to me. He felt lonely, prone to tears and was unable to enjoy time with friends. He felt it more in the night, while driving alone and when he feels that his loved ones are ignoring him. Five sessions of hypnotherapy were done in 2 months. The first 3 sessions were devoted to stress reduction, and suggestion to remove depression and sadness, which did not benefit him much. So in the next sessions he was guided under deep hypnosis to the origin of his problem. He went to a lifetime in England in the 1970s, as a young man named Alex. He is leading a happy life with his wife and three small children below 5 years, whom he loves very much. One night when he is in bed, some robbers wearing masks enter the room and shoot him. While he is dying, he is worried about the family and feels sad and lonely. Reliving that life and disconnecting from its emotions got rid of his depression and sadness and he became cheerful.

Asthma

Asthma is a chronic problem, for which an effective remedy is not found in the conventional treatments. Hypnotherapy has been used successfully in asthma patients. More than 90% of asthma has its origin in a past life, where past life regression therapy has been able to give complete relief.

> Madhavan, a 58 year old businessman came to me, in February 2016, with breathing difficulty and tightness and pain in the chest. He had initially come for a solution for a bowel disorder; once that was cleared (described in the next section), he wanted to address his breathing problem. He had asthma from childhood, which was controlled by traditional medicines. But wheezing started about 6 months back and he developed an unknown fear. Tracing back to the origin of the problem under deep hypnosis, he first went to some childhood incidences that generated fear and helplessness, accompanied by tightness in chest and breathing difficulty. Releasing the feelings from there gave only temporary relief from his chest pain and asthma. When he was stressed the problems returned. He came back after one year, seeking a permanent solution for his asthma. Under deep somnambulistic stage I asked him to go to the origin of the cause of his breathing problem; he regressed back to a life as an agriculturist. His farm is near a forest; 8–10 people are working for him. He described himself as a 25 years old man, supervising the work of his helpers on the farm; the year is 1885 and place is Maharashtra, India. Suddenly a tiger comes from the forest and all the farm hands run away, leaving him alone to face the tiger. He is scared. The tiger attacks him, mauling him on the throat, chest, sides, and hips. He feels the chest being crushed and is suffocated. There is nobody to help and he dies. After reliving that incidence his asthma and pain and tightness in the chest were gone.

Sometimes a person passes through several lifetimes till resolution is found, as was seen in the case of the elderly lady, described in chapter 9.

Bowel Disorders

Irritable bowel syndrome (IBS) is a complaint for which clients seek my help. This is a body symptom with a strong emotional basis, high stress and anxiety being the triggers in most cases. Usually the person feels a lot of tension, mostly self-created or imagined, and feels an urge to go to the toilet, which becomes almost an obsessive need that it starts affecting the normal life and daily activities. The person feels shame and suffer from inferiority feeling and starts withdrawing from group activities and hesitates to travel or plan programs with family and friends. Hypnotherapy is found to be very effective in treating IBS; releasing anxiety and building self-confidence and teaching the client to relax resolves the problem. The case of a 23year old student, who suffered from IBS, which was successfully treated by hypnotherapy, is cited in Chapter 6.

Some other bowel disorders include chronic indigestion, acidity and ulcers.

> Madhavan, the 58 year old businessman, mentioned in the previous section, had acidity and flatulence for the last about 30 years. When he burps, acid fluid came up with gas, the intensity of the discharge increasing when he is in a negative mood. Then he felt anger and irritation in the throat, pain in the chest, breathing difficulty and lacrimation. His doctor said that the sphincter muscle valve in the stomach is partially open, which brings up the acidic fluid with gas. There was a nodule in his throat, which was surgically removed, which cured his throat problem. But chest pain, acidic burps, and breathing difficulty were still there. Medicines were not of much help. That is why he thought of hypnotherapy. After 4 sessions, acidity and throat problem were relieved. He still felt chest pain and difficulty in breathing, which were successfully treated by past life regression (described in the earlier section).

Thus, in many clients, after the initial problem is resolved, the client gains more confidence and trust in hypnotherapy and brings up other issues which they want to remedy. In the present case, even though the client came with a desire to get rid of his bowel disorder, the successful outcome prompted him to use hypnotherapy to overcome other problems, like asthma and chest pain which he was suffering for many years; this is a great advantage of this treatment approach.

Diabetes

> Senthil, 50 years, a law graduate, working as Manager in an educational institute, was suffering from diabetes for the last one year. He believed it is hereditary. His gall bladder was removed two years

> back. Under deep hypnosis he was miniaturized and guided through suggestions to the pancreas and asked to describe its condition. He saw the cells week, dull in color and not secreting insulin. He talked to the cells; they were unhappy, as the blood vessels are clogged, and the blood flow is blocked. They felt sad. After releasing the emotional feeling, the block in the blood vessels was flushed out and the blood flow resumed. The cells were feeling better and healthier. Next session was done after 3 weeks. He was asked to go into the pancreas and observe the condition. He found the cells healthy, strong and bright in color and happy and functional. His blood sugar came down and is remaining in the normal range since then.

According to hypnotherapy concept, diabetes is a physical condition created by holding back of negative emotions like grief that get internalized and stored in the modern memory. Repression and accumulation of such emotions lead to the pancreas holding back the secretion of insulin (see Chapter 6). Suggestions, given under hypnosis, helps in releasing the pent-up emotions, clearing the mind of the negative energy and removing the block in insulin secretion, leading to cure. Even though the emotional release can be fast, physical recovery can take time, as the cells have to change the old memory and establish a new association, creating new neuro-pathways in the brain.

Hypertension

It is a very common problem found in people above 40–45 years. Most of the clients who come to me with hypertension are on medication, which is taken throughout life to keep the blood pressure under control. In many cases hypertension develops as an offshoot of some emotional disturbance and can be successfully treated by hypnotherapy.

> Suguna, a housewife of about 50, came to me seeking help in controlling blood pressure. She is happily married and has two grown up children who are married and settled. She has been on allopathic medicines for some years and her blood pressure remained at 90/150. Her doctor said that it could be her normal level, so it cannot be brought down. She agreed for hypnotherapy. During the interview she said that she remains tense most of the time; trivial things like visit of a family member, even her own mother whom she loved to be with, increased her tension. After two sessions of

hypnotherapy, in which suggestions to reduce tension and build confidence were given under hypnosis, she became relaxed and her blood pressure came down to 80/130. After that she went on a pleasure trip with her family to Hyderabad, where she climbed up to the top of the Charminar Tower. She was expecting her blood pressure to increase, which did not happen, and she stopped the medicines. Now, 5 years after the hypnotherapy, she is maintaining normal blood pressure without any medicines.

Obesity

Uncontrolled increase in body weight is becoming a point of concern these days. In many cases over-eating and unhealthy food habits, sedentary lifestyle and lack of exercises are causing obesity. It can be corrected through suggestions given under hypnosis. Those who take high calorie food can be helped to change food preference to low calorie and healthy food items through guided imagery. Even one session of hypnotherapy has been able to successfully change the food preference.

> In one of my classes, the demo subject was a 50 year old medical professional, who could not refrain from fried food items. However she tried to change her food habit, after a few days she returned to her favorite dishes. Under deep hypnosis, I did a guided imagery in which she was led through two situations: in the first situation she ate fried items and felt uncomfortable and guilty; in the second situation she imagined herself eating vegetable salads and steamed food items (what the client wants, information collected during the pre-induction interview) and feeling comfortable and happy; then gave suggestion to emphasize the benefit of the change in food and reinforced it by repeating the suggestion. After that session she was able to stick to her changed food preference.

Some obesity develops as a side effect of some medicines or when a long habit of smoking is stopped. Many clients who are on anti-depressant medicines are found to have a tendency to put on weight, especially in the abdominal and hip areas. These can be controlled, to some extent, by regular exercises, Yoga practice and diet control.

Obesity may also have its origin in childhood or a past life, where regression therapy is found to be effective.

One of my clients, a lady doctor, had a tendency to put on weight which does not have any connection with her eating or any other known reason. In search of its origin, she regressed centuries back to a life in a forest area, as a man belonging to a primitive tribe. There was a landslide and flooding of the river. As he runs for safety, he takes refuge in a cave. But the cave gets flooded, blocking his escape route. He sits on a rock above the water level, waiting for it to recede. But he dies of starvation before the water recedes and his last thought is that if he had been fatter, he could have survived for some more days and escaped from there. In this life that memory prompted her to maintain an obese body. Even though hypnotherapy did not make her slim, it helped her to trim down and mentally accept a healthy perception of herself.

Skin Problems

Other than infections and physical injuries, several skin problems like acne, pimples, dis-coloration, psoriasis, some allergies, etc. are found to have an emotional basis. Stress has a major role in triggering some skin reactions that are expressed as physical symptoms. Especially in teenagers, emotional disturbances and related stress are found to cause skin problems like pimples and acne. Suggestions given under medium trance, even under self-hypnosis, have been able to reduce the skin reaction; in some cases stress reduction alone gave miraculous results, even one session producing pronounced changes.

Psoriasis is a skin problem in which medicines are not found very effective and need to be taken for long, and there can be unpleasant side effects. Hypnotherapy has been successful in treating psoriasis.

Praveen, a retired Bank employee, was suffering from psoriasis for more than 10 years. He was treated for 5 years with Ayurveda medicines, which gave some relief. Then he switched over to Allopathy, which was stopped after 3 years, as his blood sugar was elevated. For the last one year he is on homeopathy medicines. It gave temporary relief and the problem got aggravated during the cold weather. So he approached me to see if hypnotherapy can help. There was severe itching and discoloration of the skin on the hands, legs and back, more pronounced on the knees and elbows. Now he had pain in the joints and was feeing sad. Six sessions of hypnotherapy were done between December 2019 and February 2020, then temporarily stopped due to lockdown. There is considerable improvement; itching and skin discoloration are significantly reduced in most areas, now noticeable only on the left knee. He is feeling happy and optimistic about the positive outcome and is eagerly waiting to resume the treatment.

Severe conditions of psoriasis may need several sessions and 6–12 months to get the full effect. I tell this to the clients before starting therapy, but most of them discontinue treatment when they see some improvement.

> A middle aged man had come to me with severe psoriasis. He had severe itching on the neck, head, hands and legs and scaly exfoliation of skin when scratched. I explained the course of therapy and told him that he has to be patient, as it may take one year or more to complete the treatment and he agreed. After 4 sessions the itching stopped, skin became clearer and the exfoliation noticeably reduced. Then he discontinued treatment.

This is the state in most clients who have consulted me for psoriasis. In some cases, psoriasis may have deeper lying causes, coming from a past life. Here regression therapy is used to go to the root cause and resolve it from there.

Surgery

> One of my clients, Ammini, an 85 year old woman, was to be operated for rectal cancer. Due to the possibility of complications, the surgeon had ruled out general anesthesia and decided to do the surgery under local anesthesia. She had some apprehension when I saw her but was willing for hypnotherapy. Three sessions were done during the week before the operation, in which suggestions were given to condition and desensitize her to the pain and promote smooth and fast recovery, the last session done 2 days before surgery. The surgery went off smoothly; even though she was aware of everything, she did not feel any pain. The post-operative recovery also was smooth and painless.

Apart from reducing pain, hypnosis can be used in anesthesia, alone or with conventional anesthetics, which helps to reduce the dose of the anesthetic. Hypnotherapy also helps to reduce bleeding in surgery and accelerate the healing process and recovery. The therapist has to spend time with the patient before surgery to build rapport and make him/her feel comfortable with the therapist and has to be with the patient during the surgery. If it is not possible for the hypnotherapist to be with the patient, similar benefits can be obtained by doing the sessions before surgery and conditioning him/her through suggestions under hypnosis, as seen in the above example.

There are published reports supporting the benefit of hypnosis in difficult surgeries that require time, as the hypnotist can maintain the hypnotic state as long as the surgeon wants to complete surgery, without the use of chemical anesthesia; the patient remains relaxed and wakes up without any effect of the anesthetic. Even open heart surgeries have been done successfully under hypno-anesthesia.

Cancers

Usually cancer patients do not come to me in the early stages of the disease, when hypnotherapy can heal, or given along with conventional treatments like surgery, radiotherapy and chemotherapy, can accelerate the recovery. Patients are referred to me mostly in the terminal stages when all other options are exhausted. In very advanced stages, where the disease has spread to different parts of the body, hypnotherapy may not be able to effect healing but can reduce pain and discomfort and improve the quality of life, as discussed earlier.

In patients undergoing radiotherapy and chemotherapy, hypnotherapy helps to reduce the side effects and make the treatment less traumatic and more acceptable, improve treatment outcome and enhance the post-treatment quality of life. A preliminary study by the author has shown that the side effects of radiotherapy could be reduced or even eliminated by hypnotherapy; several sessions may be needed, starting before and continuing throughout the duration of radiotherapy.

> Ammini, the rectal cancer patient mentioned earlier, underwent 5 weeks of radiotherapy of the abdominal area after the surgery. The general side effects of radiotherapy of digestive organs include diarrhea, vomiting, lack of appetite and weight loss. Hypnotherapy was done to control the side effects – three sessions before starting and one session each week during the 5 weeks of radiotherapy – in which suggestions highlighting the positive outcome and accepting the therapy without the side effects were given. She completed the radiotherapy without any major side effects like diarrhea or vomiting or radical weight loss.

Chapter Thirteen

Other Areas of Application

Hypno-birthing

Smitha, a 25 year old working lady, was afraid of what she had heard of delivery pain. As her due date was nearing, she approached me to see if I can help in reducing the pain. I told her about hypno-birthing, which is a method of easing delivery by reducing pain and discomfort. Through suggestion under deep hypnosis, the client is desensitized to the feeling of pain, at the same time maintaining the muscular contractions normal, making the experience a pleasant one. It was not possible for me to be present in the labor room during the delivery. So we scheduled 3 sessions of hypnotherapy during the week before her due date. She went into deep hypnosis and responded very well to the suggestions. I gave suggestion to remove anxiety and control pain to a comfortable level, at the same time maintaining the physical body functions normal, so that muscle contractions needed for pushing the child continue in the normal way. I also did guided imagery, taking her through the course of delivery, starting with wheeling into the labor room, as the contractions increase she feeling a pleasant anticipation of seeing her child, filling her with joy and love for the child, to hearing the first cry of the child, feeling proud and fulfilled as a woman and mother. This process, repeated in two more sessions, worked so well that she was mentally relaxed and calm and did not experience major pain or discomfort during the delivery.

Hypno-birthing is used in several Western countries and USA for painless delivery, where the hypnotist remains with the woman during the delivery. The hypnotherapist has to spend time with the client before the date of delivery to build rapport and expectation, and then during the delivery. Guided imagery is often used; use of triggers and anchors is found to be very effective. In case the therapist cannot be present during the delivery, a few sessions done before the delivery can achieve the same results, by a process of conditioning through suggestions under hypnosis, so that the client accepts the delivery as a pleasant experience, as was done in the case of Smitha. Subconscious mind has the power to separate emotional and physical feelings, so it is possible to address the emotional feelings without affecting the physical sensations and movements, which property is taken advantage of in hypno-birthing.

Dentistry

Shobha, a 57 year old housewife, was suffering from dental decay and pain for some years. The Dentist had advised extraction of the affected teeth, which she was postponing, as she feared the pain and discomfort it may cause. Now the damage had progressed to such an extent that there was no option other than removal of the teeth. So she approached me to reduce her anxiety and fear. Three sessions were done in 4 days. In the first session, suggestions were given under hypnosis to release tension and build confidence. Second session was done after 2 days, in which suggestion to control pain and discomfort of extraction was given. This was followed by guided imagery, in which the entire process of extraction from waiting in the dentist's office, sitting in the dental chair, feeling relaxed and calm, extraction of teeth, to recovery, getting fitted with the new denture, feeling happy, satisfied and proud of her new look, was visualized. This was repeated in the 3rd session, done the next day. Her teeth extraction was smooth and painless; it was a lengthy process, as there were several teeth to be removed, which was done in batches on different days. She remained relaxed and calm during the whole course and did not feel pain or discomfort during the recovery period also.

Dental problems are increasing these days. Several factors like lifestyle changes, food habits, tobacco chewing, poor oral hygiene, etc. contribute to this increasing trend. Some of the treatment processes, like tooth extraction and root canal treatment, cause severe pain and discomfort since most of the time only local anesthesia is used. Moreover, the patient is under a lot of stress and has a low threshold for pain. The patient also suffers pain during the recovery period. This creates anxiety and fear of dentist, especially in children. Even in adults, the thought of going to a dentist produces tension, anxiety and fear. A survey by the British Dental Association has shown that a large number of patients feel stressed and anxious about a dental appointment.

Use of hypnotherapy in dentistry was first reported in Egypt more than 3000 years ago but lost its importance as chemical anesthesia came into practice. The USC School of Dentistry in USA has been offering formal training to Dental professionals in clinical hypnosis for many years now. It is an effective method to reduce anxiety and remove fear. It can produce good analgesic and anesthetic effects. Suggestion incorporated under hypno-anesthesia helps in keeping the patient relaxed and comfortable, so he/she feels no pain or anxiety during and after the process. Hypnotherapy can also help control the bleeding, retching and gagging and reduce the trauma of a difficult dental surgery. Even suggestion given under a light trance has been found to work wonders in soothing the nerves of the patient. A couple of sessions prior to a dental appointment can reduce tension and fear and keep the patient relaxed. A study in Stockholm indicated that hypnotherapy before surgery can help reduce anxiety and minimize the post-surgical use of analgesics.

Palliative Care

Pain relief is an important part of palliative care. Those who suffer from acute pain often lose all logic and act irrationally, exhibiting intense anger and frustration, may become abusive of the family members and caretakers, and even the doctors and other health workers. The following case is an example of how hypnotherapy can help such patients.

> Jonathan, in his early 40s, is the only bread winner of a small family, including his young wife and two school going children. He was admitted in the Palliative Care Centre, Trichur, Kerala, where I do hypnotherapy on the patients referred to me. He had spinal injury and for the last one year he was confined to bed, unable

to stand up or walk around. He was getting severe headaches frequently, which made him lose all control. When he was in pain, he got angry and shouted at everyone, his wife, children, doctors, nurses, whoever is there.

When I met him, he was very depressed and pessimistic, had lost all hope in life, feeling worthless, often talking of suicide. He told me that there is no hope of recovery, he is a burden to his family, and it is better to die. I first talked to him in conscious state, relaxing him and instilling hope of recovery. He said that he loved his wife and children, but the pain in the head is intolerable and makes him mad; then he forgets himself and shouts at them using bad words. He wanted relief from the pain, as pain killers were not helping much. He was willing to be hypnotized. I used progressive relaxation and he readily went into deep hypnosis. I asked him to imagine the pain as an object, a symbol of the pain, and get rid of that symbol, the pain leaving with it. As the symbol disappeared, he felt comfortable. Then I gave a suggestion to reinforce the effect and remain relaxed and calm and brought him out of hypnosis. On waking up, he was an entirely different person, smiling, and said that he is feeling comfortable in the head and has hope for future. Thereafter I met him two more times in 3 months, but he did not need hypnotherapy; he was cheerful and optimistic, completely free from the pain.

Palliative care is an area where hypnotherapy has a lot of scope, individually and as a complementary modality. Patients under palliative care include those who are in the terminal stages of diseases like cancer, and those who are severely handicapped and unable to manage themselves, due to damage to brain and spinal cord, stroke, paralysis, accidents, etc. and need constant care. Apart from pain, they suffer from anxiety, low moods, sadness, hopelessness and helplessness, frustration, irritation, anger, depression, insomnia, feeling worthless and a burden to the family, even entertaining suicidal thoughts; many of them suffer from pain and stiffness of joints and limbs. In such cases the aim is to reduce discomfort and improve the quality of life by boosting their morale and preparing them to accept the situation and use the available remedial resources to get the best out of the situation. Hypnotherapy gives effective and lasting relief from pain, reduces anxiety, depression and insomnia, bringing hope and optimism and improving the quality of life and accelerates recovery.

> Kala, a 37 year old woman, had lost the movement of the lower limbs after a brain tumor surgery. She was depressed and sad when she was referred to me. Although not educated beyond middle school, she is very talented, writes poems and does handicraft work, but had lost interest in such things. Three sessions of hypnotherapy were done, in which suggestions to release depressive feelings and to boost positive attitude were given. She became more cheerful, started writing small poems and her interest in handicrafts was revived.

Physiotherapy

Used with physiotherapy, hypnotherapy has been found to ease limb movements and accelerate physical recovery.

> An elderly gentleman, in his late 50s was coming to the Palliative care center and taking physiotherapy for stiffness of the right shoulder and hand. He was not able to lift his hand; as the movement caused intense pain, he found it difficult to do the exercises. The physiotherapist referred him to me. Under deep hypnosis, he was asked to miniaturize himself and enter the area of his pain and view the condition. He described the problem as three nerves lying twisted and causing the pain. I suggested that he straighten those nerves, which he did, and he felt the pain reducing, finally disappearing as all the nerves became straight. After waking up he was excited that he was able to lift up the hand above his head to its full extent.

In patients with partial body paralysis undergoing physiotherapy, hypnotherapy with guided imagery and positive visualization has been found to accelerate recovery of the limbs. But it is a gradual process and will need many sessions. Physiotherapy done under hypnosis is found to produce faster results.

Geriatrics

With the increase in longevity, this century is seeing a rise in the number of old persons, along with an increase in age related health issues. In a nuclear family set up, with the younger able bodied persons living either in distant places or abroad and busy with their life, there is a dearth of helping hands. The elderly people, ranging from 65 to 85 years, suffering from different diseases and nobody to look after them, often depend on domestic help or other hired caregivers; they feel lonely, abandoned and betrayed by children, and often sink into depression; fear of diseases and death may start haunting them. Many of them also suffer from different health problems like joint pains, body pain, diabetes, hypertension, cardiac problems, restricted ambulatory capacity etc. that add to their mental and emotional distress. They find life meaningless and a burden to their children and other relatives and start fostering death wish. Hypnotherapy can help them to relieve pain and get rid of the negative thoughts and depressive feelings, find a purpose to life and positive things to do, restore optimism and the will to live.

Chapter Fourteen

Applications in Children

The doorbell of my clinic rang, and I opened the door to find a cute little girl of 7 or 8 years looking at me with a shy smile and a little wonderment in her eyes. She was Ansia and had come with her grandmother. I had met the grandmother a few days back while waiting for the train in the railway station. She was sitting next to me. The train was delayed, and we introduced each other and got talking. In the course of the conversation she asked me what I am doing. When I said that I am a counsellor and hypnotherapist, she told me about her grandchild and took my phone number. She said that the child was scared of darkness, afraid of sitting alone in the room or going near the window after it becomes dark. Later she called me and booked an appointment. Ansia said that in the night a ghost comes and stands behind the window and frightens her. I used a simple technique of eye fascination to hypnotise her and asked her to imagine herself in her favorite holiday spot. She saw herself on the beach, picking up shells and running after small crabs and playing with the waves. Then I asked her to sit down on a bench on the beach and imagine the ghost standing near her and describe it; she saw it as a woman in flowing white gown, with large protruding teeth, red round eyes and long, sharp finger nails. I asked her to imagine the ghost changing into smoke, then fill that smoke into a bottle, seal its mouth and throw the bottle into the sea and let it sink into the depths of the sea and disappear, taking away her fear. Only one session was needed to get rid of her fear. After some days, her grandmother informed me that now Ansia is not afraid of darkness or sitting alone in the room; she even volunteers to close the windows in the night.

Fear and anger are the most common problems for which children up to 12 years are brought to me. Other problems include bed wetting, antisocial behavior, lying and stealing and poor concentration and study habit. The main problems reported by children in teens are stress, anxiety, anger, study problems, lack of concentration, fear of examination, stage fear, depression, lack of confidence and strained relations with parents. Less common issues include smoking, drinking, drug abuse, porno viewing, mobile addiction, obsessive compulsive disorder (OCD), suicidal thoughts and attempts, masochistic behavior, etc.

Critical Years of Mental Growth and Behavioral Development

School age and stages of puberty and adolescence are the most critical in human behavioral development. Ages 5 to 15 are very crucial in the formation of basic behavioral pattern and can be called the formative years of human behavior. This is the best time to inculcate good habits and motivate them positively. Parents and teachers have a significant role in molding them into responsible citizens and good human beings, motivating, guiding, supporting, and correcting them where needed.

Influence of Family on Behavioral Development of Children

Behavioral development of children is strongly influenced by the people they interact with, how they are treated and the environment in which they grow up. Family atmosphere and interactions have a crucial role in the healthy development of the children. In the modern family set up, along with the increasing influence of mobile phones and social media in the personal life of individuals, quality interaction and communication among members of the family are becoming almost nonexistent. This is leading to tension and misunderstanding or lack of understanding, affecting the normal functioning of families, creating more and more dysfunctional families, where mistrust and competition among members lead to jealousy, anger, quarrels, and lack of constructive communication. Children growing up in such families do not get the love and care they need for healthy development. They feel insecure and develop different behavioral problems. In such cases, in addition to treating the child, the entire family including parents and siblings may have to be included in the treatment for effective and lasting results. Family counselling can help in releasing tension and establishing communication and bring understanding and harmony, creating a congenial atmosphere for the child to grow up.

Adarsh, a 13 year old boy, studying in the 7th standard, was brought to me by his parents, with the complaint of stealing and lying. He is an active child, is in the Tennis team of the school. He is a good student and teachers like him. He used to take money from mother's purse without telling her and she ignored it. Once on a tournament tour from school, he stole money from another student and was caught, and it became a serious issue. Adarsh is the only child of his parents. After school he plays tennis for 3 hours and reaches home tired. Both parents are employed, and they do not spend time with him. Father does not hug him or hold him, which he desires; he does not feel close to his father. He was not very communicative, was sitting and crying. Mother said he sometimes cries like that at home also. I hypnotised him and asked him why he takes money instead of asking his parents. He said that he wants to buy his favorite food from the school canteen. He is afraid that his parents will scold him if he asks them. I asked him to imagine going to a place he likes. He imagined himself on a plane going to a big restaurant near a beautiful lake. He ate Pizza and then played for some time after which he sat on a bench near the lake. A big swan comes and talks to him, asks him why he is stealing money; he says he wanted the money to buy his favorite food from the school canteen. He is afraid of asking his parents, so he takes it from mother's handbag. But he takes only the price of that food item, that also 2 or 3 times a week. The swan says that his parents love him and are happy to give him money for his genuine needs, but he has to ask them since they do not know what he wants. So from now on when he needs to buy something, he should be asking his mother or father and they will give the required money and they feel happy and proud of his truthfulness. He should also ask permission of the teacher to go to the canteen and he agreed. The swan said he is a good boy, and he thanked the swan, got on the plane and came back. Then a hypnodrama was done, in which he was asked to imagine he is ready to go to school and he asks his father for money to buy his favorite dish and he gives it happily. Now he is in the class and it is the recess. He asks the teacher for permission to go to the canteen and she allows him to go, he buys the food and eats it; it tastes much better than it did on earlier occasions because today he had asked his father and got the money. He feels happy and decides that he will always ask his parents if he needs money and be a good boy because his parents love him and are proud of him and he also loves them. After waking up he said he is happy and hugged his parents. I also counselled the parents to spend more time with their son and find out his small desires and take care of them and asked his father to occasionally express his love by hugging and holding his son close and show that he cares for him because the boy is at an age when he needs father's attention. After that session he stopped stealing money.

It appears that he was craving for the parents' attention and was doing something that they were sure to notice; stealing was his way of attracting their attention to him.

Even though clients up to 18 years only are considered as children, in my experience some youngsters behave like children even up to 21–22 years. Therefore, I follow a similar approach in such clients.

Sam, a 21 year old boy was brought to me by his grandfather. He found it difficult to concentrate on studies and had depressive feelings. He was studying in a place away from his parents and grandparents, staying in a hostel. He was more attached to his maternal grandparents than to his own parents. During holidays he preferred to go to the grandparents' house rather than to his parents, because he found the atmosphere in the parent's house stressful. He has an elder brother who is working abroad. So he had no one at home to share his feelings. His parents were always quarrelling and his mother depended on him so much that he started to feel it a burden, at the same time he was feeling guilty that he is not able to help his parents, especially the mother. He was under constant stress since he was 14 or 15. The strain was telling on him and he was going down in his studies. Five sessions of hypnotherapy, in which stress reduction, release of guilt feeling and depression, building self-confidence, motivation, and concentration were done, and his personality changed totally; he became cheerful and confident, with strong commitment to his studies and goals.

Children brought up in a dysfunctional family atmosphere are the most adversely affected, due to the fact that they do not get proper care, emotional support or guidance from the adult members; they may get blamed for small lapses or even for mistakes of adults, becoming the scapegoats. In many families where both parents are employed and do not spend time with the child, or where the parents are always arguing and blaming each other, children do not feel free to express their feelings or discuss their problems with the parents for fear of getting scolded or ridiculed. The parents feel guilty and compensate with monetary and material rewards, fulfilling every wish of the child. Such children grow up with mistrust, insecurity and inferiority, develop anger and resentment that are suppressed, leading to intolerance and lack of concern for others, manipulative of parents, siblings and even friends, antisocial or criminal tendencies and may end up to be problem children. Children who are victims of emotional and/or physical abuse get demoralised and lose confidence and self-esteem, which may lead to development of anger and resentment and mistrust of adults.

Hypnotherapy is effective in treating such children; the therapy can take many sessions, and co-operation and participation of parents are necessary for the success of therapy.

Child Hypnosis

Many children feel scared of the therapist and will not be ready to talk to him/her. The child may have been taken earlier to counsellors and other behavioral therapists, who treat the child on the basis of what the parents have said, without listening to what the child has to say or how he/she feels. This creates in the child's mind an impression of adults as bad people siding with the parents, and the therapist, being an adult, belongs to that category. For success of hypnotherapy, the child should have complete trust in the therapist. Therefore, rapport building is the first and most important part of the pre-induction interview. Small children may have apprehensions because of other experiences with hospital visits for inoculations and immunization injections. Moreover, a hyperactive child may have been warned by the parents that if he/she does not behave properly the doctor will give injection with a big needle. So the child looks at the therapist with suspicion and fear.

It is the responsibility of the therapist to build a good rapport and create trust in him/her, even if it takes more than one session.

Generally rapport building is rather easy with a child. Children are very good at imagination and they live most of the time in a fantasy world and they believe in what they imagine and say. When talking to the child, I am attentive to what he/she has to say and refrain from contradicting or criticising or laughing when the child exaggerates things, even though the parents say that he/she has a habit of telling lies; I try to go with the child so that he/she accepts and trusts me as a friend and well-wisher. When there is conflict between the parents and the child, I stand with the child, because it is what he/she perceives that matters in hypnotherapy and what needs to be addressed. It also helps in building rapport, because you change the 'bad adult' image of the therapist that the child may have into a 'friendly adult' who understands him/her. Then the child will go along with you and accept your suggestions.

Some teenagers, who may have been getting so much negative inputs from parents, teachers and other elders, build a defense around themselves and come with a defiant attitude. Sometimes a teenager may try to shock you by an unruly statement; this is a defense mechanism that they have adopted to protect their ego. As the therapist, I try to remain noncritical and non-judgmental and accept the child as he/she is. This helps to break down the defense and he/she will be ready to open up and cooperate, which is necessary for the success of the therapy.

Methods of Induction

Children are very visual and their eyes tire easily. So visual aids like pendulum, crystal ball, pen light etc. work well in small children. I have found story telling an effective technique in children up to 10 years, as they easily identify with the fictional characters. You can bring animals, birds, butterflies, fairies, etc. into the story and treatment also can be done as a part of the story. As children live in a fantasy world, they can imagine anything and what they imagine becomes their reality. Most children have high imaginative power and accept the suggestions easily, as their analytical faculty (conscious mind) is not fully developed.

> Ammu, a 9 year old girl who had undergone corrective surgery for club foot was brought to me by her mother. The doctor had advised her to practice walking with the feet pressed flat to the ground. She felt pain while pressing the feet down and therefore

> tried her best to avoid the exercise. I used storytelling and took her to a beautiful garden, where she plays with the butterflies and then a big butterfly comes to her with a special pain balm and applies it on her feet, fanning with its wings and the pain goes away and she feels comfortable while walking with her feet pressed down. She thanks the butterfly which flies away, and she returns to the room. On waking up I asked her to walk with both feet pressed down and she comfortably walked, feeling no pain.

Above 10 years hand levitation can be used for induction and then deepened further through suggestions. With children above 14 years, it is advisable to test the hypnotisability and get their consent before taking them into hypnosis. While hypnotising children I ask one of the parents to be present in the room. But some children above 15–16 do not agree to that. Then we can call the parent after the child is under hypnosis. But it is essential that the parents do not talk or interfere with the proceedings. In a case of a 14 year old boy, both parents were sitting in the room while I was treating the child. Every time I asked the child a question the mother interfered and answered it, saying that he will not tell anything on his own. So I had to send her out, letting only the father remain there; she left the room angry and in tears.

Children up to 10–12 years can be hypnotised without them knowing it.

> A 9 year old boy, who was brought by his mother for anger control, told me that he does not want to sleep. It seems that his parents had told him that I will make him sleep. I told him that he does not have to sleep, but I want to test his concentration and he agreed. I made a round mark on the wall in front and asked him to stare at that point with full concentration because I want to know how long he can maintain the concentration. As his eyes started tiring, I gave a suggestion that he is relaxing, and his eyes are closing and will close when I say 'deep sleep' and he went into deep hypnosis. After releasing anger, when I woke him up, he said with a smile that he did not sleep and heard everything I said. Session was done in the presence of his mother, so he was comfortable.

Simple techniques like eye fascination or staring at a point, with suggestion, work well with children of that age.

Emotional Problems

Anger and fear are the main issues for which children under 12 years are brought to me; other problems included bed wetting, hyperactivity, lack of concentration, and a few cases of lying and stealing. One or 2 sessions are enough to remove the problem. The case studies included in this chapter can elaborate on it.

> Regi, a 9 year old boy was brought to me by his parents. He is the eldest of three children, the younger ones are girls, aged 7 and 4. He is very short tempered, explodes at the younger sisters, even hurts them physically, and shouts at parents when angry. There was no reason known to the parents for his behavior. Regi told me that when the younger sisters disturb him or take his things, he gets angry, but he loves them and want to be a good brother to them. I used story telling for hypnosis induction. Under hypnosis, I asked him to give his anger to an animal that he dislikes. He imagined his anger transferred to a monkey which started jumping angrily, grinding its teeth and producing weird sounds. I asked him where do monkeys live and he said, *'in the zoo'* (many of today's children living in big cities have seen them only in the zoo and do not know their natural habitat). I said that we will send the monkey to the zoo and he agreed. So he called the zoo authorities who came with a big cage and took the monkey with them, all in his imagination, and his anger left him. After that one session Regi became nice to his sisters and parents and his anger was fully under control.

Sibling jealousy has been found to cause behavioral problems in children, expressed as anger, mostly in the elder child, especially when there is 5 years or more difference in age between the two children.

> Ankur, a 9 year old boy was presented with uncontrolled anger. He has a brother, six years younger to him. His behavioral problem started after the second child was born. He felt that after his brother came his parents loved him less. The mother's behavior also contributed to it. Some examples the boy cited to show that his mother did not love him as she loved his younger brother included: mother fed his brother with her hand, but when Ankur asked to be fed like that she laughed and said that he should eat by himself as he is big now. Moreover, his brother was allowed to sleep with their

> mother, but she denied that privilege to him and sent him to the grandmother's room to sleep. He felt rejected and sad, which came to be expressed as anger, first towards his brother and then towards the mother. Anger was released in one session, followed by a suggestion that he loves his brother and is caring for him as a responsible elder brother. I also counselled the mother to treat him as a child and give in to some of his innocent demands. His problem was resolved with that one session.

Even though the parents have to give more time to the younger child, who needs more care, they should be careful not to create an impression of being neglected in the elder child's mind. Moreover, some parents/grandparents do not allow the elder child to come near the baby or touch it for fear of hurting the baby. This can create anger or hatred towards the new member. This is because a child which was getting all attention from the parents till the arrival of the second child considers the newcomer as a rival competing with him/her for the parents' love and attention. Sometimes, with the arrival of the new child, some parents expect the elder one to behave with responsibility and discrimination. The child does not understand the parents' behavior and becomes confused and reacts by getting angry and creating tantrums, the only way they know how to get the parent's attention. In fact, the parents should prepare the child, much before the baby's arrival, to accept the newcomer as a friend and companion, to receive love from and give love to and a welcome play mate. After delivery instead of keeping him/her away from the newborn with reprimands, they can allow him/her to participate in its care giving small responsibilities, but under their supervision. Parents should also be careful not to do or say anything that can rouse antagonism towards the baby. In such cases, in addition to treating the child, I also counsel the parents, which has yielded good results.

> Venu, a 10 year old boy, was presented with lack of concentration and confidence. I asked him to explain his problem, he was almost inaudible. Parents said that at home he speaks normally, but in school he does not speak. He was afraid of everything, but mainly street dogs. His father said that, when 6 months old Venu was in his lap, a big dog kept its paws on him and he got scared. I used staring at a spot on the wall, with relaxation suggestion for hypnosis induction. He went deep. Then I asked him to imagine himself in a place of his choice. He saw himself in a beautiful garden in front of

a palace. Some children are playing cricket there, they invite him to join them. Then the children take him inside the palace where he meets the queen who asks about his fear. She takes him to a kennel where different types of dogs are kept. He plays with a small pup and is not afraid, but he says he is scared of street dogs. So the queen takes him to the street; there are many dogs, and he feels scared. He takes a big balloon and fills his fear into it and sends it to the sky where it merges with the clouds and disappears. He feels good. He again goes near the dogs, growing big and the dogs becoming small and scared of him and they run away. He is no more afraid and feels happy. He comes back to the palace with the queen, have meals with the king and queen and their children. There are different types of sweets and fruits and he is enjoying every dish. He thanks the king and queen, says goodbye to the children and comes back. Then I gave a suggestion that now he is confident and bold and is able to study with concentration and go out on the street without fearing dogs. After waking up I asked him to go out. There was a big street dog near the gate, but that did not bother him, and he passed by it. His problem was resolved in 2 sessions.

Fear is an often encountered problem in small children; fear of darkness and fear of ghosts are the common ones. Many children develop fear of ghosts after hearing stories or watching it on the television (as in the case of Ansia, given in the beginning of this chapter). As the stories show ghosts coming out in the night, it becomes associated with darkness. Such fears may also be instilled by the adults, when they try to control a hyperactive child by the scare of ghosts. Then the child starts imagining ghosts, giving them an image, usually human figures seen in the movies or created in its mind.

Avin, 10 years old, in 5th standard, is an only son; father is engineer, mother works in a Bank. He is a good student, and active in extra-curricular activities also and plays tennis. He is living with his father; mother is staying in another town where she is working. When I asked him what his problem is, the child said that he is scared of darkness, sitting in a room or going upstairs alone in the night, had fear of ghosts and fear of snakes. Two sessions of hypnotherapy were done: first releasing fear of ghosts and second session, fear of snakes. He was asked to imagine in a place he liked, and he saw himself on the beach. He saw the ghost as a woman in white dress, with large protruding teeth and blood dripping down from the teeth. I asked him to imagine the ghost turning into smoke, and then fill it into a balloon and send the balloon to the sky, where it collided with a big cloud and merged with it and disappeared and his fear of ghosts left him. In the second session also he imagined himself on the beach, saw the snake in the sand, and as suggested by me, caught it in a net and threw it into the sea and made it disappear deep to the bottom of the sea. That got rid of his fear of snakes also.

His father had also complained that Avin plays with toys, teases his younger cousins and is wasting time, which he should use for reading newspaper. I counselled the parents to spend more time with the child, stop criticising him for small things, give him emotional support and make him feel secure, and let him play with toys in spare time as he is at an age when playing is natural. After some days, his father informed me that Avin is happy and now moves in the house without fear, sits alone in the room and studies.

How a sentence spoken by the adults can affect a child's behavior is demonstrated in the following case.

Sanju is a six year old boy, highly active and very talkative, studying in the first standard. His elder sister, 4 years older, also studies in the same school. Sanju liked to go to school and play with his friends there. One day when he came from school, he was very upset and silent. When parents asked, he said he does not want to go to school. They did not give much attention to it. Sanju developed fever by the night, which was controlled by medicine. After that day he refused to go to school, saying that there is a tiger in the school which will eat him. His mother went to the school and talked to the class teacher. The teacher said that Sanju always talks and disturbs the class and it is difficult to control him. When asked to keep quiet, he stops for some time, but again starts talking. In exasperation, that day the teacher told him if he disturbed the class again, she will lock him in the room with the tiger. Now he is scared that if he goes to school he will be put in that room and the tiger will eat him. Any amount of assurance by the teacher that there is no tiger there and he is very safe and cajoling by the parents could not convince him. The child had not gone to school for the last three weeks when the parents approached me.

When I asked where the tiger is in the school, he said there is a dark room under the staircase (the place where the cleaning materials like disinfectant solutions, mops, etc. are stored) and the tiger is there. I told him that we will get rid of it and then he can go to school and play with his friends. I asked him to close his eyes, relaxed him, and let him imagine he is in the school. He was scared. I said I am going to arrange to send away the tiger and he agreed to my suggestion that we send it to the zoo. So he was asked to imagine the zoo authorities coming and taking the tiger away with them and he felt happy; then he and the teacher examined the room and found no tiger there and his fear was gone. On waking up, he said he will go to school and he started going to school from the next day. The most interesting part came the next week when the family visited the zoo. There was a tigress with 3-4 cubs. Sanju pointed to one of the cubs and said that is the tiger he had sent from the school. Such is the power of children's imagination which can be made use of in resolving problems.

Bed Wetting (Enuresis)

Bed wetting is a habit where the bladder empties automatically during sleep, without the child being aware of it at that time and realizes it only on waking up in the morning and finding the bed wet. Children can be toilet trained at 2-3 years of age; the child will be able to tell the parents and control their bladder. Bed wetting usually stops by 3 years of age; in some children it may take 1-2 years more to stop completely. If it continues after 6 years of age it should be considered a problem and treated.

A 9 year old girl, Anagha, an only child, was brought to me by her mother. They are a happy family, both parents are loving and caring, and there were no known emotional or other problems. She was hypnotised by staring at a point, with accompanying suggestion, in presence of her mother. Under hypnosis I asked what is bothering her in sleep. She said she is scared; in the night, the toys come near her and frighten her (she has many toys, which are kept in her room, which is adjacent to her parent's room. During daytime she happily plays with the toys, so her revelation under hypnosis came as a surprise to her mother). When I asked her if she wants the toys to be removed from the room, she said 'yes.' I made her visualize her mother removing them and she felt relaxed. She did not want anything to be put in the place of the toys. (Her mother removed all the toys the same day and the child never again asked for them). Then suggestion was given to release fear, followed by guided imagery, taking her through the process of going to sleep in the night, waking up when the bladder is full, going to the urinal, and coming back to the bed and falling asleep, to waking up in the morning feeling happy to see the bed dry and cozy. Second session was done after two days and the guided imagery was repeated, which resolved the problem of bed wetting.

I also ask the parents to set some rules for the child: child is not allowed to drink water or any fluid after dinner and is made to urinate before going to bed in the night and immediately on waking up in the morning.

Reasons for bed wetting vary from child to child. It can be caused by fear, anxiety, feeling of insecurity, trauma, even hostility towards parents or caretaker and, in some cases, underdeveloped bladder tone. If it is an emotional problem like anxiety, fear, etc. it can be released under hypnosis. If due to underdeveloped bladder tone, it may be corrected medically or through physical exercises and Yoga. Emotional insecurity is found in children whose parents are always quarrelling and do not give quality time to the child, or the child is a victim of verbal, physical or sexual abuse; then I desensitize the child to the feeling of trauma associated with the abuse. I also counsel the parents to give love and support to the child and make him/her feel secure and protected. Emotional traumas from death or separation from parents can also cause bed wetting; especially in a child who had stopped the habit, but suddenly restarts it at a point, the traumatic experience, and the resulting insecurity feeling, acts as the trigger to revert back to the earlier behavior. Releasing the trauma under hypnosis and instilling happy feeling resolves the problem.

Children brought to me with bed wetting mainly fall between 5 and 10 years. Only two cases of older children have come to me.

The oldest child whom I treated was Siva, a 13 year old boy from an orphanage. He was poor in studies, had feeling of inferiority, and every night he was wetting the bed. He did not know it until he woke up in the morning. So he was made to sleep separately on a mat, while other children were given mattress to sleep. The children used to make fun of him. and he developed inferiority feeling and became introvert. When I talked to him, he said he was scared of ghosts. Under hypnosis, he described the ghost as a dark gigantic figure, with big eyes like round red balls. He was asked to imagine it being converted into smoke and filled it in a big balloon and tied the balloon to the wing of a bird, which flew up with the balloon and disappeared into the sky and his fear left him. Then a suggestion was given to build confidence. Three more sessions were done, one session in a week, with guided visualization of getting up and going to the urinal and after emptying the bladder coming back and sleeping soundly and waking up in the morning, happy to see the mat dry and feeling proud that he has control over his bladder movements. After two sessions the frequency of bed wetting reduced to 2 or 3 times a week and stopped completely after the fourth session.

Study Problems

Most of the teenagers are brought to me with the complaint of poor study habits and lack of concentration. Study habits can be improved and concentration and confidence can be increased through suggestions. Time management is an important part of inculcating good study habits. I often ask the child to make a timetable for the daily routine and studies that he/she can follow. Under hypnosis, when I give the suggestion to improve study habit, I include the timetable in that. I have found suggestions given under hypnosis, followed by visualization using triggers and anchors (see Chapter 7), is very effective in increasing concentration in studies. In most children, two to three sessions give the desired results.

Even when the child or parent presents poor study habits as the problem, many a time, during the interview the real problem turns out to be something else. Many teenagers are confused, unable to decide what they want, lack confidence, and suffer from anxiety and fear of failure and coming up to the expectations of the parents.

Mohsin, 16 years, studying in 10th standard, was brought by his parents, father in business and mother a housewife, with poor study habits and fear as the presenting problems. He is an only child. He was away from home, staying in a hostel since he was 12 years, and recently came back to live with parents. He is finding it difficult to adjust in the new school; he is shy and timid, has no confidence, unable to make friends, has fear of talking to people, fear of ghosts, spiders, etc. He gets angry with his mother because she keeps blaming him for everything. When angry, he feels sad and cries. Five sessions of hypnotherapy were done in one month. Desensitization to fear was done in the first session and his fear was reduced. In the second session, anger towards mother was released and suggestion to increase confidence was given. After that session he was able to control his anger and make friends with other students. In the third session his fear was released, and he became more active, mingling with other children and taking part in school activities. The next two sessions were devoted to improving study habits and his problems were fully resolved.

I also counselled his mother to refrain from unnecessarily criticising him and be more considerate and understanding, in view of the fact that when he needed the parents' care and support he was made to stay away from them, in a hostel environment in which he felt alienated and insecure. During the pre-induction interview he had said that the other children used to tease him, and he used to get angry and beat them, they also used to beat him, but the warden did not help him.

Many children do not study regularly, postponing everything to the examination time and then they find it a burden. They also spend a lot of the time at home watching TV or on mobile phone, playing video games, chatting, etc. Too much use of mobile and internet and video games is found to disturb concentration in children.

Rita, a 16 year old girl, studying in 11th standard, was not able to concentrate on studies. She studies only when the examination pressure is on her. She wants to study 4–6 hours daily. Now she is spending hours on mobile phone and watching TV. She was also not able to control her anger. Four sessions of hypnotherapy were done. The first 2 sessions were devoted to increasing concentration and reducing time on TV watching and mobile use and she was able to study daily with concentration and cut short her time spent on mobile and TV. Anger release was done in the next 2 sessions, which included age regression and her anger was also controlled.

Examination fear and anxiety are other reasons which affect the performance level and grades of even a studious and intelligent child.

Usually the parents, who bring the child, have many complaints against the child, sometimes assumed or heard from someone else. Teenage children, between 13 and 18 years, are passing through a difficult period. This is a period of development when changes are occurring at the physical, physiological, psychological and emotional levels. They are experiencing the changes that are inevitable in the process of leaving the childhood and entering the adulthood. They want to show that they are grown up and can take independent decisions, but at the same time feel insecure, perplexed about what they feel in the body and mind and are overly self-conscious. They are impatient and intolerant, cannot accept criticism or advice from adults and turn to the peer group, friends, relatives of same age, etc. for advice and help in decision making. They feel that their parents, and adults in general, do not understand them and become irritated and aggressive, or introverts and non-communicative. The parents also do not understand why the children are behaving like this, and reprimand them, even restricting their movements and interaction with their friends, blaming their friends for the child's behavioral changes. This is an age when visual media has great influence and when they get addicted to mobile phones, alcohol and drugs, sex videos, etc. which distract them from their studies, and the parents may not be aware of it. Hypnotherapy has been found to be very effective in helping such children.

> Murali, a boy in his late teens, with poor study habits, was brought to me by his father. He had failed in most subjects in his 12th standard Board examination. His father said that he studies for many hours, locking himself in his room, but during the examination he is not able to recall what he studied. I talked to the boy alone and he said he is addicted to self-masturbation; when he is supposed to be studying, he usually will be watching blue films on his video and masturbating. He wanted to get rid of the habit and was ready for hypnotherapy. The cause was traced back to childhood, where at the age of 7 or 8 he was sexually abused by an older man and when he was 13, he and his friends got into watching some videos and then he got into the habit. After three sessions of hypnotherapy he got rid of the habit and started studying.

While treating these children, it is beneficial to counsel the parents also, to give emotional support and feeling of security to the child and refrain from unnecessary nagging and blaming, while having an eye on what they are up to when they sit alone locked in the room and create trust in the parents so that they will feel free to discuss their problems with them. Some parents say that they never deny anything to their children and do not interfere in anything they do. This is also a dangerous trend, which can lead the children into undesirable, even dangerous, companionships and habits.

Sometimes parents judge their children in comparison with other children like cousins, classmates, even siblings, which can demoralize the child. It is to be understood that no two persons are born alike; even identical twins may differ in certain characteristics. Different children exhibit different talents and interests, so judging a child on the basis of comparative performance in a particular field or subject is unfair and can be counterproductive.

Some young people get addicted to mobile phones and suffer from withdrawal symptoms when parents take away the facility.

> One 19 year old girl, who was brought to me by her father, was in such a state. She was found talking on the mobile for hours together, till late in the night, neglecting her studies and had got into some unsavory alliance. So her father took away her phone. She was extremely angry with her parents, shouting and misbehaving with them. The parents took her to several psychologists and psychiatrists and finally came to me. She told me that she can live without food, but not without her mobile phone. As she was adamant and did not co-operate, I could not do anything to help.

Children in their teens are also found to go down in studies as they develop romantic relations that they want to hide from parents, which creates stress. Sometimes such relationships can lead to circumstances in which the children take hasty decisions against their own interest, upsetting their studies.

> Shivani, a 17 year old girl, who is a bright student, completed her 12th standard and had cleared the entrance examination for a course in Alternative Medicines and was waiting for the admission. She had got involved in an affair with a man of 30, an Auto driver, and ran away with him without telling her parents. The parents registered a missing complaint with the police, and they traced the couple in a remote village in another state after few days, where he had taken her and introduced her as his wife. As she was a minor,

the police arrested the man and she was returned to her parents, which infuriated her. She became angry and rebellious, not eating or bathing or talking to parents. It was then the parents brought her to me. They said she has got admission in the professional course, but she missed the pre-admission counselling and her admission in the current year has been cancelled. She was non-communicative in the presence of the parents. So I sent them out and talked to her calmly, and she told me that she loves that man and wants to marry him and move out. I said it is fine, but she has to wait till she completes 18 to get married and asked her what she is going to do during this one year. She did not have an answer. Then I broached on her studies and her life at home, relations with parents and her younger sister (whom she loves but had not talked to her since she was brought back). She said she loves her parents and sister, and they are loving and caring, but they do not approve of her relation with this man whom she loves and she was feeling guilty that he was arrested by the police because of her. When I asked her about his earlier affairs with other girls (this man had befriended some other teenage girls from well-to-do families, promising marriage and cheated them), she said he has promised that from now on she will be the only woman in his life. Then we talked about her future and desire to become a doctor and how she is going to achieve it once she marries this man, as the course is expensive, and the parents are not going to support her. The man she wants to marry was earning about Rs. 8000.00 a month and will not be able to find the money for her education. Moreover, with that earning she will not be able to give a good life and education to her children in future. Then I told her that if she completes the course and becomes a doctor, and then marry, she will have a good earning that will take care of the needs of the future family. I asked her to go home and think about it and come back after 2 days. She came with her parents on the third day. She was more cheerful, was taking interest in daily activities and talking with parents and sister. She said she wants to study and become a doctor before getting married. I asked her what she is going to do if her lover comes and asks her to marry him after one year when she completes 18. She said he has to wait till she completes her course, which was 5 years from now, and if he is not ready for it, he can marry someone else. She seemed to have grown more mature and confident.

In such cases, what I do is try to buy time, as advise or arguments are not going to help. In the case of Shivani, by the time she becomes a doctor, with the respect and standing in the society for the profession, she is most likely to review her past attachment in a different angle and take a wiser decision about her future, rather than the impulsive reaction she had shown when the parents objected to her love relationship.

Mini, an 18 year old girl of 12th standard, had got into a love affair with a young man living near their house. Recently her father was transferred to another place and he moved to the new place with family and she got admission in a school there. Her lover was against it and he was asking her to go back and threatening her father on phone. She had arguments with her father and one day she left home to meet the young man without telling her parents and the issue went to the police. This had affected her studies. She wanted to leave her education and marry her boyfriend and settle down. But he did not have a good education or consistent job. His family was also not well off. Hence the parents were worried about her future and brought her to me.

In the first session I counselled her, and she became convinced of the importance of studying and getting a good job before thinking of marriage, as the man of her choice was not in a position to financially support a family. She wanted to get admission in the Medical course and sought my help to improve her grades. She was not able to concentrate on her studies and time management was also a problem with her. I asked her to make a timetable, allotting time to different activities of the day, including studying, from waking up in the morning to going to sleep in the night. Three sessions of hypnotherapy were done in one month. In the first session, after taking her into hypnosis I gave suggestion to improve study habits, including the timetable and she started studying according to the timetable. But she had difficulty in remembering what she studied; she had examination fear and her confidence was also low. In the next 2 sessions, suggestions to increase concentration and memory and build confidence were given and desensitization to examination fear was done; she was able to study with concentration and was free from examination fear. Then she said she did not want to continue the love relationship and wants to be free from that attachment. So cord cutting was done; she felt free and her relationship with parents also improved.

Some children find study boring and are not able to sit and study continuously for more than a few minutes.

> Abhiram, 17 years old, studying in 12th standard, wants to become a software scientist and wants to study 10–11 hours daily. When he was brought to me, he was unable to study even for 1 hour a day. He finds study boring and feels sleepy after studying for a short time, especially in the night and in closed room. His sleep is disturbed, he suddenly gets up in the night and cries out. He also had anxiety. I asked him to make a timetable, marking the time for daily studies. Four sessions of hypnotherapy were done. In the first two sessions I gave suggestion to improve study, incorporating the timetable. Next session was done after 2 weeks. He was now able to study without feeling bored or sleepy. In the 3rd session stress reduction and release of anxiety were done and he started sleeping well in the night and getting up in the morning refreshed and was comfortable studying sitting in the room. Fourth session was done after 2 months. He said he is studying well but has tension about examination and was not confident. So tension was released and suggestion to increase confidence was given. That resolved his problems.

Sometimes, apart from counselling parents, the therapist may need to talk to the teacher, as they may not be convinced about the change in the child.

> Anish, a 16 year old 11th standard student, found it difficult to sit and study continuously for more than 40–45 minutes. He was also cutting classes and was short of attendance. He could not control his anger; when angry he reacted violently, throwing and breaking things. His father is in Gulf and Anish is living with his mother and elder sister who is a graduate student. His mother is not able to control him. He had already broken the television set and mobile phone when he was brought to me. Three sessions of hypnotherapy were done in one month. Anger release was done in the first session, replacing it with happy feeling, which controlled his anger and violent reactions. In the next 2 sessions suggestions to improve study habit, increase concentration and time management were given and he started studying according to a timetable and with concentration. At his parents' request, I also talked to his school Principal, who agreed to adjust the attendance deficit on the condition that Anish attends the classes regularly without fail during the remaining part of the school year, which he accepted. That resolved his problem.

Some children exhibit fear of examination and anxiety about coming up to the expectations of the parents; some parents set targets, e.g. 95% in the Board exam, which can act as a stressor in many children. This information comes out when I talk to the child alone, in the absence of parents. In such cases, in addition to improving study habits, I desensitize them to the feelings of fear and anxiety, replacing it with confidence and happy feeling. I also counsel the parents to support the children and encourage them when they try to improve, instead of pointing out the short comings and blaming them for small lapses.

Some parents expect miraculous changes in the child after one session of hypnotherapy.

> A 16 year old boy was brought to me by his mother, with the complaint that he does not study at home and obtained below average marks in the class exams in several subjects. He was in 10th standard and only 2 months were left for his Board exam. When at home, most of the time he is watching TV or sitting idle doing nothing. When I asked him what he wants to achieve, he said he wants to pass the exam with above 80% marks, and he can achieve it if he studies 4 hours a day. So I asked him to make a timetable for his daily routine, marking out 4 hours daily for studies. Under hypnosis I gave a suggestion to improve study habits, including a guided imagery of his studying according to the timetable, with concentration and interest. The next session was fixed after 1 week. When he came for the second session, he said now he is able to sit and study with concentration one hour at a stretch, whereas earlier he was not able to concentrate even for 5 minutes. His mother was still complaining that he is not studying, even though she agreed that he is more serious now and sits and studies more than earlier. The boy got angry with the mother saying that she can only see his defects and not his effort and improvement. I counselled the mother to be more patient, appreciate his effort to improve and encourage him. One more session was done to improve study habits and increase concentration and that resolved his study problem.

Some other behavioral problems that can be treated by hypnotherapy include obsessive compulsive disorder (OCD), antisocial behavior, including criminal tendencies, addiction to narcotic drugs, sex videos, etc., but are less often referred to me, possibly due to lack of awareness.

Hypnotherapy is effective in treating OCD; early stages are easier to treat. But usually they are brought after other methods are tried and failed, and the clients are in their 20s, when the obsessive habits are established as a part of the behavior. Still it is possible to change the behavior pattern, but it will take many sessions. My clients, though few, when brought to me were between 22 and 30 and were on medication for 5–8 years. They are branded as sick, so even after the symptoms are controlled, parents and others do not let them come out of the stigma of being a mental patient.

> A young man of 26, I treated successfully, took 6–8 months to come to normal behavior. When he came, initially his symptoms included repeatedly washing hands (sometimes 100 times), fear of contamination when sitting near strangers in the public transports, fear that someone will take his money, using abusive words on Gods and Goddesses, feeling that someone is touching him, restless and not able to sit and study or do any work, unable to travel alone or handle money. He lacked confidence and was suspicious that people are making fun of him. The first few times his father had brought him. After 6–7 sessions of hypnotherapy, his hand washing reduced to 3–4 times, he started travelling alone in bus and was able to handle money and started preparing for PSC exams.

But his mother, a school teacher was not ready to acknowledge the change, comparing him with his elder brother, who is an engineer and working abroad. Such attitudes of parents can create obstacles in the progress of recovery. They have to appreciate and encourage the positive changes in their child and help him/her in maintaining it.

Many parents when they first notice an aberrant behavior in the child ignore it, because they do not recognize it as a problem that needs help. They take the child to a professional only when someone else points it out or it becomes severe. In some cases even a professional gets confused about the diagnosis.

Babu, a 17 year old boy, who was brought to me, was being treated for OCD, but to me it looked more like a case of mild autism. So I asked the parents to take him to NIMHANS, Bangalore and get his condition assessed and it turned out to be autism. Some of the symptoms like repetition of a particular action look similar in both conditions. So diagnosis based on one or two symptoms can go wrong. I do not treat autism, as according to hypnotherapy concept, it is a condition that the soul has opted in this birth for the purpose of learning and evolving (see chapter 1).

Addictions to drugs, sex videos, etc. are not brought to therapy in the early stages as parents are often not aware that their children are into such activities. Even where the children are caught red handed, the parents often try to hide it. Only when it becomes a nuisance that they think of taking the child to a counsellor or therapist, mostly when they are young adults. That is also one reason we rarely get such children for therapy. Vigilant parents can detect them at the initial stages when hypnotherapy can correct the behavior. Most such teenagers would have had bad childhood experiences that would have led them to such habits. Quarrels between parents, wife beating, father's drinking habit and creating problems at home, sexual and other abuses, constant blaming of the child, ambiguous statements and behavior of parents, etc. are some of the contributing factors to the antisocial behavior.

Antisocial and criminal behaviors usually attract legal actions, and the children end up in juvenile corrective centers. They can be helped and rehabilitated by hypnotherapy. But generally they are not brought to a hypnotherapist; even the few who are brought to me did not complete the treatment.

> Mathew, a 14 year old boy, is the youngest of three children, the elder two are girls and are working in a Gulf country. They had offered to take him with them and find a job for him after he passed the 12th standard. But the boy dropped out of school after 8th standard; now he just roams around with some friends. When the parents reprimand him, he packs a bag, threatens to leave home and the parents concede to his demands. He is into the habit of tobacco chewing and drugs, which he denies. He wants to become a doctor, but not interested in studying. One day he entered the OPD of a big hospital, posing as a doctor, wearing a lab coat and a stethoscope in hand, trying to examine patients. He even ventured to enter the operation theatre when he was caught and handed over to the police. Parents pleaded with the hospital authorities and the case was not registered. It was then they brought him to me. When I asked him about it, he said he has not done anything wrong as he did not charge the patients. I asked his father, who is a farmer, to engage him in some work on the farm, as he was not interested in studying. Then Mathew said

that if his father makes him work on the farm he will complain to the police and get him arrested for employing child labor. He was ashamed of telling that his father is a farmer; he had told his friends that his father works in Gulf. I counselled him, showing the incentive of going abroad as he desires if he studies and passes 12th standard. I also warned him that if he does illegal things and a police case is registered, he cannot get a passport or visa and it will end his dream of going to Gulf. So he agreed for hypnotherapy. But after one session he refused to come, and the parents were helpless.

As the saying goes, prevention is always better than cure. Parents have a big role in molding their children and ideally they have to be good role models and be clear and unambiguous when interacting with the children. A father who tells his son not to smoke or drink but does them himself is a bad role model. A more often noticed behavior is that the parents tell the child that telling lies is wrong, but when someone, whom the parent does not want to see then, comes to his house, asks the child to tell the visitor that the father/mother is not at home. The child is perplexed by this ambiguous message from the parent, which it stores in its modern memory and can affect his/her later behavior. But in the case of Mathew these were not the reasons behind the antisocial attitude of the boy. As he was the only boy, born after two girls, the parents and elder sisters (7 and 10 years older than him) pampered him, fulfilling all his demands, even giving money without asking how he spent it. He had got into unsavory company and bad habits, but when asked he played innocent, putting the blame on his friends; even when a tobacco pouch was found in his pocket and the parents asked him about it he said he did not know about it and one of his friends must have put it there, and they believed him. Now, even though they are aware of the truth, they are afraid of his threats and are not able to correct him. This is a condition found in many middle class families of India, where the overindulgent parents are blind to the small behavioral problems in their children and when they find out it comes as a shock to them. So, my counsel to the parents is that while loving your children, please be alert to their mental and behavioral deviations, if any, and use your authority and wisdom of years to patiently correct them through gentle advice and examples. You should realise that parents are the first counsellors and role models to the child. They would be the best counsellors only if they can be the best role models, as children are intelligent and observant and continuously learning from examples.

Epilogue

I hope that the previous pages have given the readers a fairly clear idea of how hypnotherapy uses the power of the mind to resolve deep emotional issues and heal mental and physical diseases without the use of medicines.

Hypnotherapy is a continuous process of search and learning, search into the depths of human mind and its spiritual magnitudes and the wide range of therapeutic possibilities of hypnosis. The deeper one delves into the mind, the more one is surprised by the revelations of secrets that it holds and the more humbling the experience, and the more motivating to probe deeper and deeper. As more therapeutic possibilities are unearthed, going to the cellular, molecular and energy levels, the day may not be far when man learns to remain naturally healthy and happy using the power of mind, the dream of holistic health without external intervention and disease-free life becoming a Universal reality, and just a thought away.

I wish all the readers good health and happy reading.

Further Reading

1. Austin, Valerie: Self Hypnosis. Harper Collins Publishers, India, 1994

2. Chopra, Deepak: Quantum Healing. Bantam Books, USA, 1990.

3. Erickson, Milton H.: Complete Works. Milton H. Erickson Foundation, USA, 2002.

4. Govindan, Marshal: Kriya Yoga Sutras of Patanjali and the Siddhas. Kriya Yoga Publications, Canada, 2000.

5. Hadley J. and Staudacher C.: Hypnosis for Change. New Age Books, India, 2001.

6. Jung Carl G.: Man and His Symbols. Dell, New York, 1968.

7. Kappas John G.: Professional Hypnotism Manual, Panorama Publication Company, 2009.

8. Krasner A. M.: The Wizard Within. The Krasner Method of Clinical Hypnotherapy. American Board of Hypnotherapy Press, USA, 1990.

9. Kübler-Ross Elisabeth: On Death and Dying. Mac Millan, New York, 1969.

10. Peale Norman Vincent: The Power of Positive Thinking. Om Books International, Noida, India, 2016.

11. Selye H.: The Stress of Life. Nd Edn. McGraw Hill, New York, 1978.

12. Shiva Swati: Redefining Happiness, The Light Works Publishing, New Delhi, 2012.

13. Shiva Swati: Emotional Energy Management (Improve Health and Positivity), Kindle Edition, 2016.

14. Siegel Bernie: Love, Medicine and Miracles. Rider, U.K., 1986.

15. Sohn Emily: Decoding the neuroscience of consciousness. Nature 571, S2-S5, 2019.

16. Ten Dam Hans: Deep Healing. Tasso Publishing, Amsterdam, 1996.

17. Weiss Brian: Through Time into Healing. Piatkus Books Ltd., U.K, 1995.

Index of Words

	Page Number
Abuse	45, 56, 84, 92, 98, 109, 137, 140, 148, 151, 158
Addictions	84, 106, 158
Age regression	71, 76, 78, 92, 150
Alcohol	23, 84, 106, 107, 108, 121, 151
Anchor	61, 62, 131, 149
Anger	13, 50, 52, 54, 55, 56, 63, 72, 77, 78, 84, 87, 88, 90, 91, 92, 96, 97, 98, 102, 103, 113, 114, 116, 118, 119, 120, 122, 124, 132, 133, 137, 140, 142, 143, 144, 150, 155
Animal magnetism	35, 36
Antisocial behaviour	137, 156, 158
Anxiety	20, 23, 38, 44, 49, 50, 51, 53, 56, 64, 66, 74, 84, 86, 87, 88, 90, 95, 103, 106, 117, 118, 199, 122, 123, 124, 130, 131, 132, 133, 137, 148, 149, 150, 155, 156
Arthritis	111, 112
Asthma	23, 72, 73, 74, 82, 84, 123, 124
Autonomic nervous system	29, 88
Auto suggestion	36
Back pain	112, 113, 114
Bed wetting	84, 137, 143, 147, 148, 149

Behaviour	76, 81
Bereavement	84, 96
Bernie Siegel	28, 57, 86
Blood pressure	125, 126
Body syndrome	57
Bowel disorder	123, 124
Breathing difficulty	74, 75, 123, 124
Cancer	20, 21, 22, 26, 53, 54, 55, 57, 82, 83, 97, 107, 111, 114, 115, 118, 128, 129, 133
Cataleptic	38, 39, 47
Catharsis	24, 27, 54, 83, 101
Chakras	54, 98
Child abuse	56, 84
Child hypnosis	140
Childhood trauma	31, 56, 88, 92, 121
Claustrophobia	74, 75, 93, 94
Complementary therapy	42, 81, 110, 133
Concentration	25, 34, 43, 59, 61, 65, 66, 84, 88, 89, 90, 103, 106, 137, 139, 142, 143, 144, 145, 149, 150, 154, 155, 156
Confidence	20, 23, 39, 43, 48, 49, 53, 56, 60, 61, 64, 65, 66, 84, 86, 87, 88, 89, 90, 93, 94, 96, 97, 103, 104, 105, 106, 116, 117, 120, 121, 122, 124, 126, 131, 139, 140, 144, 149, 150, 154, 155, 156, 157
Conscious mind	20, 24, 29, 31, 37, 38, 39, 47, 48, 57, 65, 72, 73, 77, 112, 141
Consciousness	10, 37, 57, 82, 112
Cord cutting	97, 98, 102, 154
Counselling	51, 81, 97, 138, 153, 155
Deepening	47, 48
Deep sleep	69, 70, 142

Index of Words

Defence mechanism	53
Dentistry	42, 83, 131, 132
Depression	20, 23, 30, 41, 43, 55, 57, 64, 74, 82, 83, 84, 87, 89, 96, 97, 98, 117, 118, 119, 120, 121, 122, 133, 135, 137, 139
Depth	37, 38, 47
Desensitization	49, 50, 78, 88, 92, 93, 94, 95, 105, 114, 116, 117, 150, 154
Diabetes	23, 53, 54, 55, 57, 72, 82, 84, 108, 119, 124, 125, 135
Dreams	32
Emotional block/burden	53, 55
Erickson	36, 59, 67
Eye fascination	136, 142
Examination fear	150, 154
Family counselling	138
Fears	23, 25, 30, 42, 49, 50, 66, 76, 84, 92, 93, 94, 145
Fear of ghosts	93, 94, 145, 146, 150
Fight-flight mechanism/response	30, 38
Geriatrics	83, 134
Guided imagery	49, 50, 59, 60, 61, 62, 78, 87, 103, 104, 107, 126, 130, 131, 134, 148, 156
Habit formation	32
Hand levitation	47, 142
Head aches	84, 116, 133
Hetero-hypnosis	60, 65
Hyperactive	140, 145
Hyper-suggestibility	37
Hypertension	23, 53, 57, 82, 84, 119, 125, 135
Hypno-birthing	120, 131

Hypnodrama	49, 50, 62, 63, 78, 92, 103, 114, 138
Hypnoidal	38, 47, 65
Hypnotisability	46, 142
Incarnation	24, 54, 72, 103
Induction	20, 36, 46, 47, 141, 142, 143, 144
Inhibition	30, 40, 41, 63
Insomnia	55, 56, 84, 87, 96, 118, 119, 133
Interpersonal conflict	49, 62
Irritable bowel syndrome	53, 84, 123
Joint pains	82, 111, 135
Kappas	36, 37, 89
Karma/ Karmic	24, 72, 75, 82
Life Script	24, 30, 75
Magic 30 minutes	70
Menstrual pain	114
Message units	31, 32, 37, 38, 47
Migraines	84, 111, 116
Miniaturization	112, 113
Modern memory	30, 31, 32, 51, 53, 56, 76, 78, 125, 159
Natural sleep	26, 37, 51
Negative emotions	53, 54, 55, 114, 125
Negative mindset	63, 64
Non-verbal methods	30, 47
Neuro Pathway	125
Obesity	55, 84, 126
Obsessive compulsive disorder (OCD)	57, 84, 137, 156
Pain relief	21, 110, 113, 132
Palliative care	67, 83, 115, 132, 133, 134
Past life regression	26, 71, 72, 104, 121, 123, 124

Pendulum	47, 141
Performance skill	48, 50, 102
Personality development	23, 84, 89, 90
Phobias	23, 49, 50, 72, 84, 92, 93, 94
Physiotherapy	67, 83, 134
Pleasure hormones	58
Pleasure-pain principle	29
Positive emotions	53
Positive mindset	54, 64
Positive thinking	20, 63, 64
Primitive memory	30, 54, 78, 94
Progressive relaxation	20, 22, 48, 110, 133
Psoriasis	23, 72, 127, 128
Psycho-somatic	52, 53, 116
Quality of life	22, 23, 74, 114, 115, 129, 133
Rapid eye movement	38
Rapport building	140, 141
Recovery	59, 67, 68, 109, 121, 125, 128, 129, 131, 132, 133, 134, 157
Regression	26, 71, 72, 76, 77, 78, 83, 92, 95, 104, 120, 121, 123, 124, 126, 128, 150
Reincarnation	72
Relationship issues	23, 62, 63, 84, 92, 98, 101
Relaxation	20, 22, 26, 37, 38, 39, 43, 48, 57, 58, 61, 65, 69, 70, 84, 110, 120, 133, 144
Repression	53, 125
Self confidence	20, 23, 84, 87, 88, 89, 90, 124, 139
Self esteem	23, 39, 53, 84, 90, 104, 122, 140
Sexual abuse	45, 98, 148
Skin problems	84, 127

Smoking	23, 33, 48, 84, 107, 108, 126, 137
Somnambulistic	38, 39, 47, 49, 58, 63, 75, 88, 95, 105, 110, 112, 116, 123
Sports performance	84, 103
Stammering	84, 104, 105
Story telling	47, 141, 143
Stress	26, 38, 43, 44, 48, 52, 53, 54, 56, 57, 64, 71, 72, 75, 76, 77, 84, 86, 87, 88, 90, 92, 95, 102, 106, 113, 114, 116, 122, 123, 127, 132, 135, 137, 139, 152, 155, 156
Stress reduction	48, 56, 87, 88, 114, 116, 122, 127, 139, 155
Study problems	106, 137, 149
Suggestibility	37, 46
Surgery	83, 93, 95, 111, 115, 128, 129, 132, 134, 141
Teenage	86, 92, 120, 127, 141, 149, 151, 152, 153, 158
Therapeutic interventions	46, 49
Time management	106, 149, 154, 155
Transcript of life therapy	89
Trauma/Traumatic	20, 31, 36, 45, 56, 71, 72, 75, 84, 86, 88, 92, 93, 94, 95, 96, 97, 98, 101, 120, 121, 129, 132, 148
Trigger	43, 56, 61, 62, 73, 76, 94, 116, 117, 123, 127, 131, 148, 149
Verbal suggestions	21, 38, 47, 48, 58, 60
Visualization	49, 59, 60, 61, 66, 67, 134, 149
Weight loss	84, 129

www.ingramcontent.com/pod-product-compliance
Lightning Source LLC
Chambersburg PA
CBHW020912180526
45163CB00007B/2704